$8 24.95

WITHDRAWN

D1129673

MY EPIDEMIC

**An AIDS Memoir of One Man's Struggle
as Doctor, Patient and Survivor**

Andrew M. Faulk, M.D.

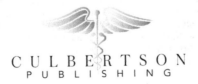

C U L B E R T S O N
P U B L I S H I N G

Cover art: TreeHouse Studios, Winston-Salem, North Carolina
Author photo: Lorinn Coburn

Poem "Memory Unsettled" by Thom Gunn is used with the permission of the Estate of Thom Gunn

Edited by Jerry Rosco

Michele Karlsberg, Publicist
Michele Karlsberg Marketing and Management
https://www.michelekarlsberg.com

Culbertson Publishing
info@culbertsonpublishing.com

ISBN 978-1-7334291-0-8 Hardback
ISBN 978-1-7334291-1-5 Paperback
Library of Congress Control Number: 2019913281

Printed in the United States of America

for my guys

MEMORY UNSETTLED

Your pain still hangs in air,
Sharp motes of it suspended;
The voice of your despair —
That also is not ended:
When near your death a friend
Asked you what he could do,
'Remember me,' you said.
We will remember you.
Once when you went to see
Another with a fever
In a like hospital bed,
With terrible hothouse cough
And terrible hothouse shiver
That soaked him and then dried him,
And you perceived that he
Had to be comforted,
You climbed in there beside him
And hugged him plain in view,
Though you were sick enough,
And had your own fears too.

—Thom Gunn

ACKNOWLEDGEMENTS

As in any project of such ambition, a great many people give of themselves. First of all I am indebted to Jerry Rosco, author of the biography *Glenway Wescott Personally* and editor of *A Heaven of Words* and Glenway Wescott's *A Visit to Priapus and Other Stories*, who provided the comprehensive initial edit as well as patient direction and technical assistance throughout this undertaking. I am greatly indebted to Anita Rachel Tierney, my good friend from my days at Columbia University, who took on the extraordinarily difficult task of transcribing the manuscript from its original handwritten form. Both Jerry and Anita gave me unflagging inspiration and heartfelt enthusiasm. Words fail me when I attempt to express my gratitude to Lorinn Coburn, who contributed remarkable clarity of thought and a profound understanding of life and relationships in ways I haven't always recognized. I am greatly indebted to Louis Bryan, Jr. and Shannon Biggs who generously gave me constructive criticism and invaluable suggestions, as well as Bob Coe, LCSW, who provided penetrating insights into the people and times of the Great Epidemic. I am also indebted to Dick A. Bretto, Linda Gromko, M.D., Billy Tyler and the late Bill Litts who contributed to my efforts through their love and unabashed partiality. Thomas M. Reich, with his striking abilities in wordplay, provided much encouragement. I am also grateful for my late brother, Stephen, and his wife, Linda Faulk, who freely gave their particular histories. All of these people, in championing the project, reinforced my determination to complete what was both a challenging and satisfying labor of love.

I especially thank Mark Higgins, M.D. and Greg Pauxtis, M.D. from whom I learned much. I also want to acknowledge the support and contributions of Lawrence Otis Graham, Joseph Dunn, Teresa Gardiner, Lynne Gaudinier-Bell, Nicola Bucci, and my cousin Gary Olsen and his remarkable wife Pat.

I wish to especially thank my late father, Ernest Faulk, for traversing what was a formidable distance in psyche and religion in order to mend a relationship and provide much inspiration and a quiet heart.

No expression of gratitude would be complete, of course, without thanking my husband, Frank Jernigan, for providing constant support and occasional remark.

Besides all those named above, I also thank my patients, many described here, who gave me their trust and intimacy, insight and instruction, and much in the way of creating not only this manuscript but also the man I am today.

ANDREW M. FAULK, M.D.

INTRODUCTION

This book is about my epidemic—a very personal experience with AIDS in which I found myself as doctor, patient, and survivor. Not only have I been infected with HIV for over 30 years, but I'm a physician who limited my practice almost exclusively to those with HIV during one of the worst periods of the epidemic: 1984 to 1991. These were years in which the only thing medicine had to offer those of us who were infected was the treatment of individual opportunistic infections and, as much as possible, a "good" death.

In spite of my efforts to separate the two roles of doctor and patient, every patient's illness became a mirror of my own disease. Every time I walked into an examination room I was seeing me, talking to me, diagnosing me—in every patient I saw, I saw myself. Throughout this period, exact statistics were unknown but I assumed I was part of the vast majority that would die relatively quickly; I had no idea that I would fall into an extraordinarily small group which appeared to live indefinitely. Of course my continuing to live defines me as a survivor.

It is my hope that this book will be a reminder of the role AIDS played in reducing the rampant homophobia with which we lived in the years before HIV. The diagnosis of AIDS forced many to come out as homosexual. With the onslaught of HIV, a change in society's outlook came, for at last we were seen as what we had been all along: fathers and mothers, sons and daughters, brothers and sisters. Society's "discovery" of our ubiquitous presence, however, came at far too high a price—but it did come. And with this recognition came the enlightenment that our sexual orientation was of less consequence than our character (to paraphrase Martin Luther King, Jr.). This book memorializes the environment which played a significant part in changing our society from one of unapologetic homophobia to gradually expanding acceptance.

I was never a researcher, so this book is about serving patients "in the trenches" and the exhaustion and heartache which came from treating those with such an extraordinarily lethal illness. During the course of my practice, I participated in the care of approximately 50 patients who died, each as different as any person is from another. Some of their stories I've told here in order to document the pride and hope, sacrifice and courage, of those with HIV and their caregivers. In every patient I attempted to supplant fear and pain with ease and serenity. And for every person I helped face death, I helped prepare myself for the same.

I continued treating immunosuppressed patients until my own disease compromised my abilities. This book records how I've subsequently carved out a life for myself which has been varied, full, and, for the most part, happy. I've lived my life largely in a sense of modified denial: I say "denial" because I live ignoring the consciousness I have a disease, "modified" for I take my medications religiously and consult my doctors with the same dedication. Others have documented this health crisis with great empathy and eloquence, but I believe there are few physicians who have stood in my shoes and written about their experiences—few infected have written of treating those infected. This is the story of my epidemic: my personal fight with HIV, my personal and professional struggles with my orientation and illness, and my endeavors to provide my patients and friends with assistance in their walk off this planet.

* * *

Since the end of my practice, I've learned that the best method of dealing with loss is not the route of solitude and silence I often chose. Occasionally in the following pages I explain that I lacked the time or energy to properly grieve—that my work demanded tunnel vision in order to be executed with efficiency and empathy. Such methods are and were unhealthy. It would have been better had I sought out supportive individuals or groups in which to process my losses and register my turmoil. But such insight was not in my emotional vocabulary at the time. It is now.

I must apologize to the great community of lesbians and straight allies who came to our aid in as varied, gritty and sacrificial ways as is possible. There's little mention of them here because my work didn't happen to overlap with their remarkable contributions. I can never express sufficient thanks, however, to this group of untiring people who gave of themselves from the very beginning of the epidemic.

Many will find the persistent use of masculine pronouns grating. During the course of my career, however, by chance I cared for only one woman with HIV and therefore the universal use of the masculine gives my notes an accuracy that a more even-handed presentation would not.

While I use literal descriptions for almost all of the people I write about, especially those now deceased, a few of my characters are composites of different individuals. In the same spirit of respect and protection, names have usually been changed.

A HANDPRINT OF THE PAST

Well, this was the way it was. Or at least the way it was for me. For there is nothing in my story that makes it any more or less accurate than those told by so many others who lived through the worst days of the epidemic.

More than 30 years after I was told I was HIV-positive, I found myself with my husband Frank, walking into a furnished house in Cazadero, California, to spend a weekend away from the routines of life. And there on the right side of the mantel was a "pinscreen," a curio consisting of a small lucite box of silver-colored metallic rods, a 3-D "executive" toy, maybe 10" X 8", designed to capture the terrain of one's face, or hand, or whatever is pressed against it. If one flips the box over, however, all the metal rods fall back into their original, shapeless configuration. Like an old-fashioned Etch-a-Sketch, this toy could create an impression technically faithful, but easily wiped away.

It reminded me of visiting the apartment of my friend Norman Nash, in the 1990s, who showed me his own pinscreen. In his, poignantly, lay the handprint of his deceased lover. It held all the turmoil and sorrow of our time. Each time we visited his apartment in Elizabeth, New Jersey, he would survey it with a sadness and foreboding. The little device was never meant to capture a likeness permanently; its charm was in its transient preservation of an image which was easily erased by merely tipping it over. "What do I do with this?" he would ask. "I can never erase it, but I can't protect it forever."

MEDICAL SCHOOL AND THE COMING STORM

During my years of medical school at the University of Washington, Seattle, in the early 1980s, I had a long-distance relationship with a New Yorker named Gene. From time to time I would fly back to New York for this holiday or that and stay with Gene for a few days. It was during one of those visits that I learned of the death of a young handyman named Jeff. This was to be the first AIDS death of a friend. Jeff had been one of those relatively impoverished men in their late 20s/early 30s who hadn't been fortunate enough to attend and graduate from college and weren't part of the class of excruciatingly handsome, gym-going, successful young professionals of the gay community. He was, nonetheless, clever, articulate, and incredibly resourceful in making a living in what could have been, for him, an overwhelmingly expensive and hostile Manhattan. He was in a group of floating men without steady income who were friends of Gene and his neighbor Joseph, an artist in the same building.

Although we weren't close friends, Jeff and I knew each other, and occasionally heard about each other through Gene and Joseph. Gene and I had once visited Jeff's apartment, and found him in the midst of writing a porn novel, not his first, an activity that supplied him some income. He also made the odd dollar installing home sound systems and producing small battery-powered, light-emitting *objets d'art* which blinked and counted with colored lights.

Sometime during those years in the early 1980s I was visiting Gene and noticed Jeff's attractive little wall art—now with its blinking lights burnt out. At the time, Joseph was in the apartment on a small errand. Seeing the art silent and dark, I asked them about Jeff. He had suddenly fallen ill, Gene reported, and had entered the hospital and died within two weeks of some poorly-defined central nervous system disease. Numerous specialists had been called in on his case but to no avail. Once Jeff had passed away, as Gene had a key to Jeff's apartment, it had fallen on him to go with Jeff's father to unlock the apartment. In a scenario that was to be repeated over and over in those years with different grieving family members in different homes, the two of them opened his apartment, and together worked through his various possessions. At some point they were both embarrassed to find sexual paraphernalia and this inadvertent stumbling into the intimate details of Jeff's life made them feel horribly intrusive. As they went through the rest of his belongings, his tearful father repeated, "I don't know what to do with these things. I don't know what to do."

During my conversation with Joseph and Gene, Joseph was initially perplexed as he had confused Jeff with Scott, another one of his friends. Scott, unlike Jeff, had drifted away from him and the first evidence Joseph knew of a problem was when he had been out in Greenwich Village. Walking down Bleecker Street, Joseph had looked up to see Scott's apartment standing empty for he had, in that same disturbing manner, died suddenly.

The three of us were thrown by the sudden death of the two men and the mysterious nature of their illnesses but we later realized it had to have been AIDS. Our anxious astonishment was based on an earlier time when such youthful deaths were exceptional, before many of us began to exhibit the emotional shut-down of a population permanently stunned and bereft of the emotional energy required for grief. Bewildered, our review of these two early deaths was a pivotal moment for me—for all of us. The epidemic had already begun its terrifying machinations and, without fully understanding, we had begun to experience the sudden and incomprehensible loss of friends, acquaintances, and neighbors.

In the beginning of medical school the long-distance relationship with Gene worked well: we saw each other at least twice a year. As our holiday reunions were infrequent, times spent together were all the more cherished. One semester I was even able to study in New York. I lived with Gene on the Upper West Side and the relationship didn't seem to miss a beat. Gene was my window on the art and literary world of Monroe Wheeler (a key figure in New York's Museum of Modern Art) while Joseph became my view into the local social world. Through him I began to hear of the groundswell, the rising number of AIDS deaths. Soon after Jeff had passed, I learned that the man whom Jeff had once paid "key money" for a loft apartment, Larry Richardson, had died. Larry had been a Broadway stage designer and was in a crowd of successful New York men.

This group of more or less successful men, whom the rest of us greatly envied, was a segment of the population that seemed particularly blessed. Born with a baseline of good looks, gym workouts for these men seemed effortless and productive: they merely touched a weight and seemed to instantly hypertrophy. Following work, they exercised, came home, had a "power nap," and raced to the bars and bathhouses at the time their more conventional peers were heading to bed. Out of the house at 11 or midnight, they socialized until 2 or 3 in the morning. And the next day they were up early doing household chores or getting to the gym before work. Their energy seemed boundless; they seemed to effortlessly juggle work, gym, social life, and the necessary daily chores of grocery shopping, bill paying, laundry, and cooking. Cleaning house was, perhaps, not performed as thoroughly as their gym workouts. (Not that there weren't plenty of anal-obsessive-compulsive men whose apartments were so spotless that they more than compensated for the untidiness of their peers.) Besides this baseline of envy, most of my brothers lived under an abiding assumption that their more socially-successful peers were having more sex, better sex than they. It's impossible to sort out how much of this was, in fact, real and how much was fantasy. The more worldly will also fault me for not taking into greater account those whose lives were routinely augmented by various pharmaceuticals.

As Joseph's wider social circle mirrored that of the gay population as a whole, the escalating death toll was increasingly unnerving. At this point, the enormity of the number of deaths began to hit those like me who had wishfully assumed that only the most sexually promiscuous and drug-addled were at risk. After this assumption was proven wrong, our next misguided urban legend—that we wanted to believe—was that the epidemic was largely limited to the "players" among us: the political and social leaders, the most successful, the most handsome, those with the most resources to travel and those with the most contact with others. This assumption, too, was quickly proven wrong.

It became clear soon enough that anyone could die from AIDS— from the successful Wall Street executive to the "party boy" to the drug-ravaged homeless. If this terrible new disease could reach any of these circles, it could reach any of us.

THE PIED PIPER OF HAMELIN

In those days, the fairy tale of the Pied Piper of Hamelin was on my mind. The story of an event which supposedly occurred in the 13th century involves a rat infestation of the medieval town of Hamelin which ended successfully when a magical "pied piper" was employed to lead the rats away from town by playing his magic flute. After the task was completed, the story goes, the town fathers refused to pay him the agreed-upon sum. In retribution, the piper played his flute again, but this time the children of the village were the prey that followed the flautist into a magical opening in a rocky mountain from which they never returned. There was, however, a cut-off point at which those farther down the procession were saved. Now, in my tragic real-world tale, there had to be a clear demarcation between those ahead and those behind. Was I at the head of the line—one who had enjoyed many sexual exploits and therefore would pay the highest price? Or was I at the end—one who had initially felt excluded, yet escaped the piper's song and lived to tell the tale? During the years that followed, my mind was to return to this image, and this question, again and again.

In the ensuing years I was to travel to New York many times, and each time the number of Gene and Joseph's acquaintances lost to this mysterious illness rose at an accelerating pace. At this point, however, although the number of dead were increasing, no one with whom I was intimate had become ill. So the terror remained, for me, at abeyance. But not for long.

In my third year of medical school at University Hospital in Seattle, I did an Internal Medicine rotation. It was then that I saw my first AIDS case, or, more accurately, witnessed its surroundings,

ANDREW M. FAULK, M.D.

which involved hyper-sanitary isolation. I didn't participate in that unfortunate individual's care, I merely saw the Attending physicians' moon-suits from a distance. The partition of the room itself was such that one couldn't see that patient even in passing. The hushed tones of the doctors involved, and the high degree of isolation—as well as the fact that we students were not allowed any part of the case—spoke volumes. There always exists doctor-patient confidentiality which, of course, is taken very seriously, but in this case the usual clipboards and chart were hidden away and closely guarded. These were such times when an AIDS diagnosis brought individual patients some hospital fame.

PROFESSIONAL SECRECY

In 1984 I graduated from medical school. I had had occasional visits to New York where I'd see Gene and my extraordinary friend from Columbia, Nita Tierney. And at the UW I had important friendships with Linda Gromko, Ron Fletcher, Connie Smith and one or two other medical students. But I didn't share the more intimate parts of my life with anyone at school; so these were, on the whole, years of loneliness.

My policy then was simple: I would disclose my sexual orientation to no one until I had safely earned every degree that I wanted. I refused to have any diploma or professional endeavor taken from me because of my sexuality; and in service to that cause, I also did not disclose to friends or casual acquaintances. During the late 1980s, in fact, there were periods of renewed prejudice in public opinion, if not legal thinking, regarding HIV-positive physicians and the doctor-patient relationship. Could patients become infected with HIV through infected doctors? Should infected doctors be allowed to practice? In 1985 California Rep. William Dannemeyer introduced a bill in Congress to prohibit anyone with AIDS from working in the health care industry. The line between homosexuality and AIDS could be difficult to grasp. Not all gay people had HIV, not all HIV-infected people were gay. To the homophobic and those less familiar with the fact HIV is spread by sex or contaminated blood, misunderstanding of the distinction was spread by politics or ignorance. Confronted with such a little-known and terrifying disease which had no truly effective treatment, didn't it make sense to do away with overlapping segments on a Venn diagram and just assume that all gay people had AIDS? After all, I didn't become Board Certified until 1987

ANDREW M. FAULK, M.D.

when the debate was at its peak. It was impossible to predict how any given institution would react to an HIV-positive physician. My ambition was profound. Would disclosure to the UW bureaucracy have resulted in termination? Probably not. I was more concerned, however, with homophobic individuals quietly sabotaging my career than any formal difficulty with the University.

Now, looking back from the safety and comfort of the second decade of the 21st century and distant from the Bible belts of America, my self-imposed isolation appears self-defeating and I review it with a certain amount of regret. The pressure of the epidemic forced personal disclosures which helped create an entirely different world after the turn of the last century. Society has changed, and I have grown wiser with age. If I had it to do over again, I believe I would be willing to sacrifice my professional ambition and take the risk of coming out. But then I quite possibly would not have been able to help our community in the ways I was.

CHILDREN'S ORTHOPEDIC HOSPITAL—
SCISSORS AND A FLASK

In my third year of medical school, I began a clerkship in pediatrics at Children's Orthopedic Hospital of Seattle. If surgery was fueled by egotistic showmanship and hypertestosterone, then nurturing oxytocin-rich pediatrics was its opposite, at least according to conventional wisdom. But interestingly enough, my experience was not to be as warm and fuzzy as most people encounter. Our teaching attendant was a Dr. LeFou who thought of himself as something of a comedian. In the long white hospital jacket of an Attending physician, he kept a pair of shears. It was his habit, I was to discover later, to suddenly produce these scissors and amputate the necktie of an unwitting student before the startled individual became aware of what was happening. He also believed that "Attending Rounds" with his students should be brief: to guarantee this routine, he offered to pay for students' breakfasts if rounds lasted less than 30 minutes. This ensured that instruction didn't take too much of his day since it naturally truncated our discussion.

The premature ending of our discussions had quite an effect on me, and my trust in the system. When I mentioned my negative assessment of the built-in system for brevity, it was one of my rare moments of confrontation and an impolitic impulse to be sure. But a few days later when we met for rounds, Dr. LeFou shocked me by brandishing his ever-present scissors and attacking my tie. The blitzkrieg of his pocketed scissors was his common *modus operandi*, and what was left of my tie hung from some inglorious threads. In logical defense I suggested that my tie could have been, among other possibilities, a family heirloom. My criticism of his maneuver made

ANDREW M. FAULK, M.D.

him all the more angry with me, for my comments on his teaching style was apparently already on his mind. Suddenly we weren't pals anymore. For someone who so easily projected his horror of castration, my reaction was unforgivable. When the gravity of his response became clear, I made light of my resistance. But his sense of humor had vanished and he, an Attending, felt disrespected by a lowly third-year medical student. He notified the school that my knowledge was suspect and my patient interaction inferior.

The administration immediately pulled me from the rotation: a report of a substandard doctor was not taken lightly. What followed was a month of sequestration and ancillary testing. My degree, my future profession, was in sudden doubt. And it had nothing to do with my sexual orientation but was based on my resistance to Dr. LeFou's castration anxieties!

It was a tough month for me. I had suffered for years from the "Yuppie Complex" of not fully believing that I deserved my position, and so feared my "impostor" status would be revealed. Those four weeks, however, proved I was more than capable of my responsibilities. But after that anxious month I understood my position in the system was far more precarious than I had ever dreamed.

Despite the restoration of my standing, I was appalled by the situation into which I had unknowingly stumbled. These were adults teaching adults—there should have been no room for the type of gameplaying to which I had been subjected. Seeing the relationship between Attending and student as something more transcendent than a game of cat and mouse, I had thought Attendings were to provide support rather than have their psychological insecurities indulged. According to the Bible, "vengeance is mine saith the Lord," but He would have no input into the slaying of this particular Philistine. In a juvenile act of revenge I am somewhat embarrassed to recount, I concocted my own retribution of fire and brimstone for Dr. LeFou. On random nights he would be awakened at 3 or 4 in the morning with a phone call for which he would, presumably, shake himself awake only to discover a disconnected phone. Should he have pursued the incidents, he would've found the calls couldn't be traced as they were placed from different hospitals in the UW system and the phones involved were accessible to a great number of hospital employees. It was regretful that he couldn't have known that this was punishment for a specific crime but, no matter, the child in me was gratified that Dr. LeFou was paying a price.

In my last year of medical school, I took the only elective offered in Virology. The specter of HIV was slowly growing and I expected competition for one of the two available positions. But after registration I was surprised to find that I was the only one signed up for the rotation. Before the age of HIV, most sites for viral testing and research were in pediatric hospitals as it was the pediatric population which more frequently fought lethal viral infections, and so it was with trepidation I once again walked the halls of Dr. LeFou's Children's Orthopedic Hospital. This time the experience couldn't have been more different. The work was largely research in a lab which had a relaxed, friendly atmosphere—the researchers had been working together for a long time and their relationships were based on shared work and shared success. The lab itself, made up of multiple booths with glass separations and safety fans, was astonishingly high-tech, and as we worked we wore white paper throw-away suits, hats and shoe-coverings as well as clear plastic goggles. Toward the end of my six weeks, I was in the most central section of the laboratory when I heard a deep resonant chime of four notes. As I was in the middle of a task, I was only half-listening as a disturbingly calm woman's voice announced: "This lab has just sustained a biologic accident. Please leave everything behind and walk to the nearest exit." I heard the same message repeated. The glass doors had already begun to shush closed when I stirred myself out of a daze and scampered to the exit. One of our most capable researchers, an endearing and shy Iraqi ex-pat, had broken a flask; alone, she had remained behind as the glass doors shut. The other researchers and I looked at her forlornly as she, wearing the white uniform which covered her body except for her goggled eyes, stared back at us with what I took to be calm acceptance before she methodically began the clean-up process.

The shattered flask had contained HIV-infected matter.

ANDREW M. FAULK, M.D.

WITNESSING A NEAR-DEATH EXPERIENCE

During my senior year as resident at what was then Pacific Presbyterian Medical Center of San Francisco (now California Pacific Medical Center, CPMC, the name I will use throughout the remainder of this book), 1986-87, an event occurred that was a direct contradiction to my personal beliefs—and perhaps an admission of a different kind of possibility. To be senior resident meant that I was supervising a junior resident and an intern who had the responsibility of admitting all patients that night who weren't surgical or didn't require immediate intensive care. By definition, this also meant that I was not responsible for those patients admitted before 5 p.m. that day. I was responsible, however, for admitting patients after 5 p.m. and running any "Codes" (emergencies) throughout the hospital, except those in the medical or cardiac intensive care units.

Sometime in the early hours of the morning a Code was called. In this case, an older man's heart had stopped and he had ceased breathing. As senior resident, it was my responsibility to reach him as quickly as possible and revive him as best we could.

The respiratory team, the pharmacy, the head nurse of the unit he was on, and I all rushed to his bed. The alarm had been sounded by a nurse as he wasn't tethered to an alarming cardiac monitor. When I reached the room the patient was already receiving CPR as others were placing cardiac monitoring patches on his chest. He was a man somewhere in his late seventies who had been admitted to the medical floor that day for some problem other than cardiac. When I walked in his room he was unconscious as he wasn't breathing and his heart had stopped beating. The nature of my duties were such that I never actually touched him, leaving it to others to perform the manual operations such as chest compressions, intubation and starting a large-bore intra-venous (IV) line. My duties were to direct the seven or eight others in the room while monitoring all the information available. Electrocardioversion—electric shock to the heart—was required at one point. It wasn't a particularly long intervention as a combination of IV drugs and cardiac compressions revived his heart, though leaving him comatose. The patient had survived, and we congratulated ourselves on a successful Code. He was transferred to the Cardiac Intensive Care Unit (CICU) and I was left to my routine obligations of supervising the physical exams and admitting orders of the interns on my team.

The next morning, as the admitting responsibilities were ending and another team took charge, a nurse in the CICU called me: "Dr. Faulk, you've got to come down here and see this for yourself—you must have run a hell of a Code!"

Sometime between 7:00 and 9:00 a.m. I found my way to the CICU and into this man's hospital bay. I was in my hospital scrubs, without my white lab coat, as the previous night's work had left me disheveled and, as I had needed to discard my lab coat, I was without my name tag. There was no appreciable difference in my attire from all the other interns, residents and nurses coming and going through his room that morning. As I parted the curtain of his bay, there was my patient, as described, sitting up in a chair and eating breakfast with his wife at his side.

Immediately upon seeing me, he turned to her and said angrily, "That's the guy, that's the one who did it to me!" Above her remonstrations I asked him what it was I had done that so upset him. "You! You were the one who brought me back, and you had no right!" He proceeded to tell me that he had been in a beautiful place, a place of harmony, happiness and unity with a benevolent world. He had been in the process of crawling into a green meadow through something like a wooden fence when, evidently with some violence, I had caught hold of him and dragged him back to the far different surroundings of his hospital room. But, I asked him, how did he know that it was I that had brought him back? Being a patient in an intensive care unit is terribly disorientating, not only because of whatever ailments produced the resulting incarceration, but also for the constant intrusion of all manner of doctors, nurses and technicians asking this or that or performing examinations and procedures. An intensive care unit, for those who aren't familiar with them, is a loud, busy, often unhappy place, where a patient receives many things, but neither rest nor serenity are among them.

I went on to question him. First of all, how did he know it was I? I knew he hadn't heard my voice before the tumultuous event of his cardiac arrest—if then. Nor had he seen me in the hours after the incident, nor before my visit to his bay that morning. The night before, had he seen me from some place above his bed?

No.

If he didn't know me by sight or voice, how could he know it was I? He didn't know how it happened, but he knew I was responsible.

Was he a religious man? Had he seen any personage such as Jesus?

No, neither. He had not been a religious man and, he insisted, this incident wouldn't change that. The only way this experience had affected him was that now he had no fear of death. He had been in a beautiful place, he told me, where he felt at one with a serene universe. I looked at him now with IVs, cardiac monitors, urethral catheter and nasal oxygen cannula, all producing a cacophony of disturbing beeps and buzzes. He looked up at me, simultaneously angry and forlorn: this was not where he had been—nor wanted to be. Throughout his denunciations his wife sat visibly disapproving of his remarks— especially those inveighing against me and my efforts. I was acutely aware of the perverse irony in the man's profound dissatisfaction with what I saw as a professional triumph. Nonetheless, he had been in a blissful place, and my "bringing him back" was reprehensible to him, and neither I nor any other doctor should ever do that to him again. The man asked me, how could he ensure that this experience wasn't repeated?

I told him a simple "No Code" written by an on-site Attending physician would mark his chart as a Do Not Resuscitate (DNR) patient.

"Then do it," he said. "Do it right now!"

I walked out of his room and telephoned his Attending physician. He would be down soon from his regular hospital rounds, but if patient X was so determined to have an immediate change in status, he'd circumvent protocol and okay the "No Code" over the phone. I found the charge nurse, and she and he spoke. I firmly believe everyone should have ultimate control over their own body, especially when it comes to issues of life and death. I wrote the order and the patient's chart was flagged as DNR.

There was no easy, rational explanation for this incredible event. Was his vision of a transcendental world of peace and unity merely the result of signals from a disrupted, dying brain—as studies consistently reproduce? Was his identification of me an indication of a presently-unknown means of communication? I can believe that science has not yet discovered all the ways in which we converse: it is not beyond the pale for other, presently unknown, forms of information transference to exist. Nevertheless we have no scientific confirmation of such phenomena. But even with some undiscovered form of human communication, to an outside "civilian" a Code is a chaotic affair. A routine Code, as was this one, would test the limits of such aptitude; with the various nursing, respiratory and pharmacy personnel, the state of their various tasks and reporting the patient's response, the room can become a baffling uproar of activity. Someone unfamiliar with this emergency event—or unconscious—could easily be perplexed not only to what was being done but also who was in charge. How would communication in these circumstances translate into an ability to connect my "transmission" with the physical me? And how could a brain suffering from oxygen deprivation activating the neural signals of death be able to identify my particular "voice"?

I have always been impressed by the education I received at the University of Washington School of Medicine. There it was taken for granted that an unconscious person had the ability to hear—and on some level understand. My irascible gentleman may have heard elements of the commotion, but to identify the individual with ultimate responsibility was a stretch. Besides, the next morning when I walked into his hospital room, he had recognized me before I had spoken or could be identified by scrub color, name tag or activity.

Once immersed in HIV care, I tried to will myself to believe in a greater cosmic structure than what I could perceive. I wished for a universe, a god (however ill-defined), that would take my dying patients into a heaven of some kind. Into some comforting afterlife—be it Christian, Muslim, Hindu, Shinto, or whatever—some serene existence without pain, sorrow or isolation. Yet in spite of motivation and this compelling involvement in a near-death experience, I can't will myself to believe in heaven. Perhaps one day I'll find it possible to believe—to choose to believe—in a higher power without the nagging

ANDREW M. FAULK, M.D.

sensation I'm fooling myself. Until then this episode, whether due to science or the supernatural, remains the most powerful cognitive dissonance of my life.

MEDICAL PROFESSIONALS—
THE WORST AND THE BEST

With no clear data on route of transmission, HIV had a paralyzing effect on the medical system, and a form of anarchy emerged. In the early years, in San Francisco, I witnessed food trays abandoned by the food and kitchen staff outside the door of patients with HIV, relatives too frightened to walk into their loved ones' rooms, phlebotomists refusing to perform blood draws on patients, funeral homes rejecting the deceased for mortuary preparation and burial.

I feel solidarity and indeed great pride with those physicians who dealt with plagues throughout history. These overwhelming times (1980s and 1990s) revealed the best in my colleagues. In the very early years in San Francisco, when so little was known about AIDS, I never saw an intern, resident, or Attending physician ever express the slightest hesitancy in treating our AIDS patients. There was no task beneath their status: our physicians, whether in training or attending, would pick up a food tray on the floor left outside of a patient's room and matter-of-factly deliver it. I have never been more proud of my fellow physicians as when, without self-consciousness or pause, complaint or question, they would perform a hundred examinations and procedures—almost all requiring the simple act of touch.

By the time I moved to Los Angeles in the late 1980s such demoralizing incidences by ancillary staff had ended and I must add that the nurses involved in treating those with HIV were of such constitution that the exposure they encountered did remarkably little to intimidate them. They were without trepidation in their devotion to their charges. Although they may have flinched from

ANDREW M. FAULK, M.D.

time to time when splashed with blood or other bodily fluids—as we all did—their speed and thoroughness in their duties bespoke a fearless dedication to the wellbeing of these patients.

A MENACE PRESENT

The post-graduate training system had matched me in Internal Medicine with CPMC in San Francisco. Internship I knew would be ghastly, with unbelievable hours of work. What I couldn't know was the upheaval that was to come.

That year of internship was one of the hardest of my life. Because of the fantastic hours of work—I once clocked 110 hours of work in one week—there was little time for friends but nevertheless I had a few. I had met Louis Bryan during my interviews in San Francisco and he became a good friend. I still had Gene Spencer, although he was a continent away. I managed to meet Dick Bretto that first year—a generous, practical man who remains a close friend to this day. But those kinds of hours didn't make for a social life and the other interns, the Attending physicians, and the nurses soon became nearly my entire social world.

Early in that year, it fell to me to do the "History and Physical" of an AIDS patient with cryptosporidium, an organism which produces life-threatening diarrhea. It was known that crypto patients in San Francisco, mysteriously unlike other locales, died quickly after the diagnosis; I knew that our patient was not long for this world. But, no matter, I wanted to do the best job possible. In an environment in which the science was so unknown, I took this opportunity to get as complete a sexual and recreational drug use history as possible. I was still living in a world in which we all wanted to believe that anything this terrible had to be brought on by the patient himself. (I still cannot bring myself to use the term "AIDS victim" although it is not far from the truth.) Surely it was some disastrous combination of drugs in concert with wild promiscuity—far outside of my harmless marijuana

ANDREW M. FAULK, M.D.

and the infrequent sex that I thought would leave me safe. I quizzed this man as thoroughly as possible. To his credit, he unabashedly answered every one of my detailed questions fully, although most were very personal, covering such subjects as recreational drug use, sexual behavior and food preferences. What exposure might he have had at work? In his home? Was he breathing fungus, pollution or bacteria? What was his medical history? Any unresolved systemic disease or infection? Had his sexual contacts been diagnosed with an immunosuppressive disease? Diseases in his family? Malignancies, infections, immunosuppression or hyperimmune conditions?

Perhaps the Attending physician sensed my feverish reach for complexities or co-factors which would make the patient stand out from the crowd of other gay men who were apparently left untouched. This history was too detailed, however, for him to be a routine patient of any type, even for a patient with AIDS. After reading my exhaustive work-up approvingly, the Attending doctor's only comment was to ask whether or not I was planning a career in research.

The patient would soon be dead and his story would have to be told through our notes. Perhaps in them, and in the thousands of other notes from the thousands of other patients, could be found a clue leading to the conquering, the extermination, of this murderous virus. My hope was that my pages of notes would speak for him after his death and his sacrifice wouldn't have been in vain.

THE WORLD TURNED UPSIDE DOWN

In the Fall of 1985, there were several days in which I found notes attached to my front door from a group wanting to interview me for a study. Cryptically there was no information on its focus, who was conducting it or why I had been chosen. When at last they knocked on my door when I was at home, I discovered they were from the U.S. Center for Disease Control (CDC) and were studying HIV. Would I take part in their study? Absolutely! I would do whatever I could to help hunt down this killer. But why my door, why me? Later I was to discover that choosing subjects entirely at random is one of the best techniques for optimum statistical accuracy. I made an appointment for their clinic and was soon answering an exhaustive questionnaire about my sexual history and recreational drug use and my blood was drawn at a nondescript site near what was then Children's Hospital. When my part in the study began, there was no test for the virus but that was soon to change.

I can no longer remember how many times I was to answer questions and have my blood drawn during the months that followed. But it was on October 2, 1985, that the researchers asked me if I wanted to know the results of the newly developed HIV test. Although I didn't realize it, I was completely unprepared for my results. I didn't think about—hadn't thought about—the repercussions of an answer in the positive. My nonchalance was testament to my certainty that I had had less sex than my peers; I was certain that I was at the end of the Pied Piper's bewitched queue, not the beginning. Such was my denial.

The test was positive for HIV antibodies: I was infected.

I had been near enough to the front of the Hamelin-piper's line after all—the mountain had closed behind me, not in front. Nothing in my life would ever be the same. I know no word that would be hyperbole in describing that terrible moment of understanding. I well remember the sensation of blood draining instantly from my face. Clinical experience wasn't necessary to know that I had been given a death sentence. I harbored no illusion that I was to survive this disease; I was as mortal as my brothers and just as there was no magic bullet for them, there was none for me. Had I received the diagnosis of any number of cancers, I believed, I would have had a more certain future: my prognosis would have had wiggle room. But that was not the case. On that October afternoon in 1985, my life was changed forever.

The researchers were well prepared. Would I like to talk with a psychologist? I felt so knowledgeable of medicine that I believed such a meeting would end up to be like me talking to myself. What would a psychologist know that I, in opposite position, would not? What could they say that I wouldn't say to a patient in a similar situation? That day I misjudged the value of what therapists have to offer. Although they couldn't have changed my status, they could have started me on the way to acceptance and developing the emotional tools I would need for the rest of my life.

Upon walking out of the clinic, I spent an hour hunting for my car. I had parked directly in front of the clinic and now its location was a complete mystery! At the age of 30, I had just been diagnosed with a lethal illness. I was certain my career was ended, that my relationships were finished and my life was over. National Public Radio was on the radio as I drove away from the clinic; it was reporting the death of Rock Hudson, the first major celebrity to die from AIDS.

I'm not sure how I managed to remain a competent physician during those first few weeks after I learned my status, but I carried the information alone, telling no one. What I, the physician, would have told me, the patient, would have been to say yes to psychological counseling for this burden was too much for any person to bear alone.

But for years I didn't tell anyone—I didn't see a psychiatrist. And for years I continued the same mistake I made that afternoon. I kept this inside; I told no one what you read here. For years after I left medicine, I mistakenly assumed that if I couldn't give answers

I had nothing to say—that the telling of my story was only valid if it could calm horror, manage sorrow or allay physical pain. Now I realize what many people have: our individual histories are rich in solace and hope, that in telling them and listening to them we exercise our humanity and that they frequently give healing where medications and treatment cannot. Now I realize that simple words strung together have the ability to provide relief where there is no remedy. That is my hope with this story of the epidemic—that it may be useful for doctors and patients in some other ordeal of plague.

I agonized over whether to end my career in medicine. Even though I had struggled for so many years, it hadn't yet truly begun. In order to become a physician, I'd calculated an academic trajectory years in advance. I had applied to Stanford every year since 1974, first for undergraduate college, then as a transfer student in my sophomore year, then for its medical school, then for its internship program, and finally for its Internal Medicine residency. I was turned down—again and again. In fact, I was to receive a rejection letter from Stanford the year following my last application—apparently my name was in their selection committee or admission computers with some permanence. I could paper a small bathroom with their rejections. Since 1975, I'd chosen college courses to facilitate entry into medical school, taking classes in the summer with weekends full of homework and concentration. Judging universities against each other is a fool's errand, but I had transferred from Georgetown to Columbia in a perception that Columbia would be a better launching pad for a medical career. Despite constructing my strategies so carefully, all my planning, my years of education and training and the years of self-denial and sacrifice were no defense against the damage that this small virus could do.

Outside of work I did nothing for two weeks as I wrestled with the impossibility of my situation. The next one and a half years of training, should I live that long, would be filled with persistent stress and crushing exhaustion destructive to my immune system. Maybe I had only months to live—was this how I wanted to spend my last days? Clearly continuing my residency would shorten my life. While I knew and respected those who live to work, I was about to discover whether that was my truth as well. At the end of those two weeks of contemplating my future, I scheduled an appointment with Dr. John Gamble, the Chief of Medicine of CPMC, in order to resign my position. It was time for me to stop living in the future and begin living in the present.

It's difficult to describe my feelings that day. Even in Dr. Gamble's office I was to remain essentially alone—I couldn't tell him that I was HIV-positive because of the possible legal ramifications concerning the patients I had already treated; this was unknown legal territory. In those dark years of the last half of the 1980s, there was public debate about the safety of HIV-infected doctors treating HIV-negative patients. It was a "don't ask, don't tell" era for HIV-positive physicians. People could suspect all they wanted, but suspicion was one thing, admission quite another. For had I disclosed my HIV status to Dr. Gamble, the gears of the legal system would have likely engaged. My HIV status could have opened the hospital to liability, even though we knew that transmission was limited to exchange of body fluids.

So instead I told Dr. Gamble that the hours were overwhelming and the stress unmanageable. I was giving up my position.

Dr. Gamble listened thoughtfully to my resignation and, instead of accepting it at face value, replied that he didn't want the program to lose me. I was one of their best interns, he responded, and he was considering the program's loss even more than my own.

"What, Dr. Faulk, do you need?"

I was incredulous—what did I need? Throughout my academic years in medicine, the ratio of applicants to positions was always so high that we knew we were expendable. Should we be unable or unwilling to perform as required, there were others who would be only too happy to replace us. But having carefully weighed my health against my residency, I wasn't prepared to consider half-measures. I told Dr. Gamble that I would need a month off. I was more than certain my request would be refused.

"What else do you need?" he quietly responded.

In all my planning I hadn't anticipated flexibility. I was astonished. What else?

The option to take another month off whenever I needed it, I said. Gamble was relentless. "And what else?" After taking a month off now and retaining the option to do so again at any time, if I could end stress whenever I wanted, perhaps I could continue my career. I could think of nothing else I needed.

His wisdom was strikingly apparent in his last question: would

I be able to finish out the day? A doctor identified as troubled to a hospital administrator was not to be taken lightly. Although stunned by what had just occurred, I said yes, of course I could finish out the day.

I started that month by lying in bed for two weeks watching TV and drinking beer—a curious choice as I don't like beer. In retrospect, I should have sought counseling, but I struggled on my own—without help or audience. I didn't even venture out to gay bars where, even keeping my secret to myself, I could have had some support. Aside from re-thinking my career, I needed to generate a new self-image: a person with a terminal illness who could enjoy whatever life he had left.

In the ensuing years when I was to deliver an HIV diagnosis to others, I would tell my devastated patients not to give up hope and that in every epidemic throughout history there were a number of survivors. Although I was always to encourage this optimism, the percentage of those who did well appeared to be incredibly small and, knowing this, I never assumed such a possibility for myself. The exact numbers may have been unknown but preliminary anecdotal results were grim. I had no expectation of survival.

ANDREW M. FAULK, M.D.

FINDING A DOCTOR FOR MYSELF

After the roller coaster descent of learning that I was HIV-positive, I had to pick myself up and for the first time in my life find a physician for me. Doctors were advertised, occasionally with photos, in the *Bay Area Reporter* (the local gay "rag"). Before contacting anyone, I investigated a prospective physician's hospital affiliation—I couldn't end up being admitted to my own hospital or one closely affiliated. I found one of the doctors well-known for excellent HIV care, Dr. Bill Owen, was associated with St. Luke's Hospital. There was a considerable wait to see him, but I would white-knuckle the delay for the benefit of being cared for by someone well-versed in HIV.

He was thorough and knowledgeable in a way that assured me that when things were looking bad, he would perform well—hopefully with brilliance. One of the advantages of being on the inside in the world of medicine is the increased sense of connectedness one feels with other doctors and staff and the lack of surprise with whatever may follow in the way of medical strategy. After that first examination it was time to get my labs drawn. I sat in a hard plastic chair at the end of a long, green linoleum corridor which smelled of disinfectant. How sick was I? My new doctor told me to wait for the lab results to return before I went home.

After 20 minutes, he walked out and informed me that he needed to re-check the platelet count. The tests showed thrombocytopenia (low platelets), which could be an early indication of HIV progression and a serious problem. Or it could be due to a simple and common lab difficulty. As I began examining myself for bruises, which would indicate inappropriate bleeding, another blood sample was taken. I sat in that hallway for another 20 minutes of waiting and then the answer came back: no, it was just a frequent lab miscalculation. For the first time I was seeing the nightmare that chronic, fatal illness would mean, the first feeling that it could well be unbearable, the first feeling that it was all simply too much. It would've been good at that moment, or at least better, if I hadn't been sitting there alone. The majority of my past relationships had ended poorly, but at this moment it would've been so much better to have another person present. I internally debated my situation; I was okay I told myself. Well, no, it was terrifying, but there were, after all, pain killers and anti-anxiety drugs, mind-numbing by either one route or another. Being a physician I could stay in the loop—as much as I wanted to be in the loop (perhaps more than I should be). But to be faced with the end of my career, after I had gotten so far. Surely the world must be playing a cruel joke on me! Often in training I had felt like an adolescent because I was always in school without an income or days off. But now, here I was, stepping off the planet before I'd had the chance to live like an adult in an adult's world.

On my second or third appointment with Dr. Owen, a writer who was doing an article on Dr. Owen and AIDS wanted a photo of him examining a patient. Would I be willing to be that patient? I was initially unwilling but thought better of it and allowed them to take a photo when they agreed to only show my back with Dr. Owen facing the camera. Although I refused to be photographed for obvious reasons, I was also feeling some embarrassment about having the disease. I've discovered that there is some amount of shame, it seems, with any disease: if one can feel it with a non-infectious "innocent" illness such as Multiple Sclerosis, then it certainly is felt in HIV. I'm not immune to such feelings, so I'm glad I never saw the photo.

The Christmas break of 1985 was the most emotionally turbulent school breaks I have ever had. As if to emphasize the mind-bending horror of HIV, through a mutual friend in Seattle I learned that a gay physician I met had developed AIDS, began living in a tent in his backyard and died after three months. This of course was nothing compared to the news that I was HIV-positive. But I was in for greater sorrow and chaos: I was to lose my major source of emotional support. That year I flew to Los Angeles as Gene had changed jobs and moved there; he, too, had been tested and was, thankfully, HIV-negative.

I hadn't noticed it before, perhaps it hadn't been there before, but Gene was now using a sing-song voice to announce the illness or death of anyone with AIDS whether they be friends, acquaintances or celebrities. It was the same tone a mother might use to say to a child "I told you not to _____, and you did it anyway." While it's difficult to describe spoken tone on paper, I have no trouble describing how it made me feel—I was alone when it came to my status. It was a stance, communicated sideways, that said those with HIV were responsible for their illness. As I was HIV-positive, his reaction to my status created a separation; before, I was part of an "us," now I became part of "them." Gene was disconnected from those of us with HIV, and over time it became more and more painful to bear. Even though we had a long history, and I loved him dearly, I ended the relationship just the same.

AIDS, sadly, unraveled some of our community's fabric as well. For even in the gay community, among a few here and there as in Gene's case, I had come to detect occasional subtle, and not so subtle, messages which signaled a psychological distancing between those with HIV and those without it. Early on there was much fear and finger-pointing in our community by those reaching for the false sense of security that came from believing AIDS was caused by use of recreational drugs—principally "poppers," butyl- and amyl-nitrite. Conspiracy theories began to pop up, such as a belief that the US Government was developing and spreading AIDS as a method of annihilating homosexuals.

Later on, when the transmission of HIV was better understood, those with AIDS were condemned for careless behavior and now-disavowed promiscuity. HIV represented sexual activity itself, and perhaps some of those HIV-negative men, as was true for some heterosexuals, believed that some pay-back, some retribution, was in order for those who were HIV-positive who had presumably enjoyed sex without restriction. And there seemed to be an element of unspoken envy in their judgement.

A communication that we with HIV were deserving of our disease was an echo of the message broadcast by that large slice of the mostly-homophobic heterosexual community unaffected by the epidemic and comfortable with any reason to condemn us.

Obviously all of this failed to take into account that all that was required for infection was one exposure to one person. Like pregnancy.

A DIFFERENT WAY OF LIVING

I now found myself with a very different *Weltansicht* from the young. Not only was I not indestructible, I could be close to dying without objective signs. Any bump or discoloration of the skin could be nascent Kaposi's Sarcoma. Any cough or tickle in the chest could be budding PCP. Any headache or simple act of forgetting could be evolving AIDS dementia or progressive multifocal leucoencephalopathy (PML, an infection in the brain). After my initial visit with Dr. Owen and the scare of thrombocytopenia, my T-cells were found to be in the high 300s. (At the time, as in so much else, we had no test for viral burden—another test helpful in determining extent of infection and/or timing of approaching illness.) This was significant as most HIV-related diseases appeared to be occurring below the threshold of 200 T-cells. But as I was to emphasize with my patients, we didn't know the exact correlation between disease and T-cell count in any one individual. As the epidemic progressed, however, we learned that the correlation between a very low T-cell count and rapid death seemed absolute. Although the long-term survival rate appeared to me to be—in my non-scientific, anecdotal assessment—10%, this survival rate didn't apply to those with T-cell counts lower than 200. If one's T-cell count was below 100, for example, imminent death was almost certain. But even this information wasn't absolute, there was the question about the status of T-cell function—that someone's T-cells might be more effective than usual—perhaps explaining the man I treated who lived nearly six months with T-cells below 50. Nothing could be absolutely certain; we were, after all, biologics.

It was about this time that I developed a small, flaky, psoriasis-like patch beneath my left eye. It was somewhat itchy but without other identifying features. From the beginning of the epidemic, most patients whose disease had progressed to full-blown AIDS had a seborrheic dermatitis—a red, flaking rash in a malar distribution: worse in and between the eyebrows, above and on the sides of the nose, and on the chin. My solitary site, about the size of a nickel, was unusual for HIV in its location but consistent in appearance with the common rash of AIDS. I over-diagnosed this area and it only confirmed what my lab tests showed—I was HIV-positive and my immune system was possibly damaged. Noticing this small lesion, as minor as it was, colored my consciousness and threw the dark, unexamined, edges of my life into sharp relief. How often had I been dishonest or unkind? How frequently was I judgmental or impatient? The disease reached into my consciousness and made me question my values and integrity. I reflected on the how, and even why, of transcending the darker side of my personality and becoming a better person.

Maybe my preoccupation would have been lessened by sharing my fear with others. However, I knew confiding in others in the medical community, as educated as they were, was tricky for it could have possibly jeopardized my career. I didn't feel I had the energy or resources to be a legal test-case for retaining HIV-positive physicians. Thoughts of being questioned about my HIV status brought back memories of being asked earlier in my life if I were gay—those answers shame me to this day. I wasn't going to repeat any attempts of deception now. It was an uncomfortable paradox of my time and situation that in my epidemic safety was found in neither admitting, nor denying, my status. It was a solitary road.

At the same time the society surrounding me was wrestling with the parallel issue of "forced outing" of gay people due to diagnoses of AIDS. I was present at bedside on several occasions, when my patients were subjected to cruel rejection by their families as they learned of their sons' diagnoses, and thus their sexual orientation. But these painful encounters eventually contributed to what was to be a huge advancement in the acceptance of gay people and our movement for legal rights. In a binary world of "us" and "them," for mainstream Americans we were "them." Yet the epidemic served an unexpected purpose: yes, we were "them," we were gay, but to the surprise of society and even a few of us, the epidemic showed we were everywhere. And once we were out and society recognized our ubiquity, people got the message that we are sons and daughters, aunts and uncles, brothers and sisters, mothers and fathers. And once everyone discovered our identities, *en masse*, discrimination would be on the path to extinction.

Few people are willing to take away the job or apartment of their gay grandson.

HIGH DRAMA IN THE CLINIC

I'll never know if the gun was loaded that day. To the onlooker it may have appeared to be uncommon courage but I was responding less with bravery than as someone already facing a death sentence.

As residents and interns, twice a week we would hold clinics during which we would treat those living in the neighborhood. It was in my last year of residency, 1986-1987, that I was supervising a psychiatry intern. Often doctors heading for psychiatry feel a little less capable in the "hard science" of high octane medicine, but an internship in medicine was necessary in order to be licensed. Robert Hauser was gay and as insecure and weighted down as any of our psychiatry interns. He was terrified at being thrown into the enormous pool of technology. Whenever I was on-call with him, I did my best to boost his confidence while paying a little extra attention to his work. On more than one occasion I had reassured him that he would do well. And when he expressed those moments of panic and futility, my message was consistent—he would get through this without problems and survive internship hell. I was Robert's cheerleader.

It was during one of these clinics that I heard a slight scuffle in the outside hall and looked up from my notes to see one of the nurses who worked in the clinic, and whom I knew well, rush into the conference room. "Dr. Faulk," she said, "we need you in the hall right away!" Although I was expecting an unconscious cardiac patient on the floor, what I found surprised me.

There in the hallway stood my insecure intern, Robert, standing stiffly and looking me right in the eye with a steely calmness I will always remember and admire. Standing in back of Robert, slightly to the side, stood a man with dark, greasy hair in his early thirties. In his right hand he held a gun pointed at Robert's back. I've never been a hunter and I'm not used to seeing guns—their appearance unsettles me. Standing 25 feet away, my eyes traveled from the gigantic gun to Robert's eyes to the disheveled man and back to the gun.

As I entered the hall, the man with the gun was talking. "Why won't you give me the Percocets? I need them and you know it!" The nurse to whom he was talking stood motionless and looked at me. Another nurse, in the distance behind, was at her grey metal desk dialing for security.

I said the only thing I could think of. "Oh, sir, we don't allow guns in the hospital—they frighten the patients."

He said he didn't care, we were going to listen to him. We did.

"I'm hurting and those sons-a-bitches aren't doing nothing about it!"

As I began walking to him I said, "You know, Dr. Hauser doesn't control pain management. I do. If you're going to aim that thing at anyone, it should be me." Now it was my turn to swallow hard as he pointed the pistol at my belly. Robert didn't move. As I reached the man I said, "You don't want to hurt anybody," and grasped the barrel, motivated in that moment by the thought that I simply didn't want that thing pointed at me. I was shocked; he allowed me to take the gun out of his hand. Security arrived, the drama ended and Robert Hauser had survived another day, a day more demanding than most. And I had been more at peace facing a potentially fatal gunshot wound than the long, tortured course of an AIDS death.

ANDREW M. FAULK, M.D.

MY YOUNGEST LOSS, TOMMY G.

I had rotations in the Intensive Care Unit (ICU) of CPMC as an intern and resident on and off during the years 1984 through 1987. It was during my internship year there that I cared for the youngest AIDS patient I ever saw. Perhaps the memories have acquired a more emotional patina than the events at the time, but I doubt it. In my early years as a physician, many AIDS patients ended up on ventilators—usually as a result of *Pneumocystis jirovecii pneumonia* which, at that time, we knew as *Pneumocystis carinii pneumonia* and called PCP for short. I was too inexperienced, too untrained, to have firm opinions on whether those thought unlikely to recover should be placed on ventilators.

Tommy Gordon was one of our earliest AIDS patients. He was particularly memorable because he was admitted to the ICU at age 17; his 18th birthday occurred there while he was on a ventilator (a machine that mimics natural breathing and so infuses the lungs with oxygen). I had not admitted him to the hospital, or the ICU for that matter, and during the entire time I cared for him as a patient I never exchanged one word with him as he was usually unconscious. There wasn't even a moment of meaningful eye contact, as he was heavily sedated and his eyes were taped shut to save his corneas from the damage of infrequent blinking. In the bed he looked small, thin and pale. He may have had visitors but I don't remember any. I heard from his admitting medical team that when he was questioned about how many men he had had sex with, he responded with, "How many days are there in a year?" He was open about his trade; he was a hustler.

Hospitalization in any ICU is a horrendous experience. In fact, the sleep deprivation and opiate medications, not to mention the severity of whatever disease process is responsible for placing them there, routinely results in an ordeal so traumatic that, thankfully, the patient rarely remembers their experience. But this, of course, does nothing to diminish the actual ordeal of an ICU stay. It may appear from these statements that I somehow disapprove of Intensive Care, but nothing can be further from the truth; I just acknowledge the trauma to the body and mind of such patients requiring this level of care. Being placed on a ventilator is profoundly disturbing which is why ventilated patients are put on strong opiates so they don't struggle against this mechanized breathing.

So there we were with this teenager on a ventilator. I wasn't alone when I debated with the ICU Attending physicians whether or not his suffering should be allowed to end by discontinuing the ventilator. We doctors in training, to the person, argued that he should be allowed to die. His family, which lived somewhere in the San Joaquin Valley, was not involved in his care. With much difficulty, his mother had been contacted. She had said that her home duties—a job and a child—didn't permit her to visit. She abdicated any responsibility for his care to the hospital's Attending doctors (who were our instructors and the physicians with the ultimately authority). In spite of our clear and persistent explanations of his terminal diagnosis, the mother's response revealed her sad state of denial along with a disturbingly blasé attitude. "You do what you think best. Tell Tommy hello and I hope he gets better fast."

The Intensive Care Attending physicians, thus given ultimate license, ruled that his life support be continued. They argued, "What if you allow him to die and a cure for AIDS is discovered tomorrow? It's unlikely but possible. How would your judgment stand then?"

Tommy Gordon died on the next to the last day of my first Intensive Care rotation. With the ICU team I had cared for him the entire six weeks, during which he remained in coma and near coma. He had not been able to speak a single word during this period, nor had his consciousness cleared enough for him to signal us in any way. His only communication, if it were indeed that, had been agitation and pulling at his IVs and intubation equipment. I looked down at him in that hospital bed, small, frail, emaciated. He was at the mercy not only of his disease but of his oblivious, apathetic mother and the medical system: a system that could neither cure him nor grant him a dignified death. It was heartbreaking.

PHONE CALLS IN THE NIGHT

Throughout my career, I always instructed the nurses caring for my patients that if they debated calling me at all, they should just call. If a medical problem unexpectedly turned into a more difficult situation, hesitating to have called me would only have made the situation worse. There was always a chance an assessment could mean nothing, but I believed that when I "signed up" to be a doctor, I wasn't just agreeing to the title but the responsibility as well. I was committed to patient care even when it began to affect my own health. It was with this understanding that I encouraged the nurses working with me to show no reticence about calling me no matter the hour. I swore to them that they would never be criticized for that call at 3:00 a.m.

To be a physician meant that one had enlisted for both the good and the bad. To me this was part of the agreement, our contract with society.

LOUIS AND ALLEN, 1987

I first met Louis Bryan in a San Francisco bar while in town in 1984 for an interview for an internship and residency at CPMC. Louis—slender, intelligent, exceptionally articulate (he speaks with just a hint of the west Texas in which he grew up)—was 43 at the time. We soon became friends. Louis' partner, Allen Day, was fair complexioned with a blond drooping mustache; he was an artist of extraordinary talent who worked in graphic design south of the city. Even though I wasn't looking to replace him, Allen nonetheless felt a mixture of jealousy and genuine dislike for me. In a way, it was no wonder as there was a chasm between my sensibilities and his—I happened to be visiting their apartment in the Castro one afternoon when Allen arrived, having just bought a pair of red tennis shoes. When asked if I liked them, I offered something non-committal. But then, not willing to let well enough alone, I let slip my true opinion with, "Well, at least they must be comfortable." This only solidified his distaste for me. In spite of this, and other unintended insults, Allen was, over time, forgiving: he allowed me entry into his and Louis' group of close friends. This was quite the largesse as the two of them would create, on special occasions, lavish evening dinner parties for which Louis would create an extraordinary variety of gourmet foods.

After these dinners, during a happy time filled with discussion and humor, when the plates still sat on the table, our hosts would produce a small, clear plastic vial of cocaine. Carefully constructed to apportion a single "dose" at a time, the squat little bottle, the size of a man's thumb, was then passed, person to person, around the dining room table. The camaraderie I felt persisted long after any transient "buzz" from the bit of cocaine I inhaled. When our friends began to suddenly drop out of sight (only to appear later in obituaries), the *Weltanschauung* of living in San Francisco in the mid-1980s gave us a permission, as if one were needed, for such "debauchery."

Towards the end of these evenings, Allen would bring out his "Retirement Fund," his portfolio of remarkable drawings. He worked in many different styles and techniques and never drew a face the same way twice. His collection was large and he believed that, when the day came for him to retire, these images would generate sufficient money, if not to live comfortably, at least to cover his needs. In the end, however, Allen wasn't to need any retirement portfolio.

But there came a time when those faces around the dining room table became fewer and fewer; somber, empty chairs growing in number until the dinners ended entirely. It was in the middle of February 1987, during my last year of residency, that Louis called me. He was anxious and upset; Allen's speech had become nonsensical and he had stopped going to work. Spending more and more time in bed in full retreat, Allen had developed a dry cough and a fever. Could I come over right away? When I arrived, I was struck by the uneasy mood in their grey Victorian house. As is so often the case in California, the contrast between the bright afternoon sunshine outside and the dark shadows within were disconcerting. I walked into Allen's bedroom and marked the difference between the gaunt form lying in front of me and the dinner party host of the past. He was emaciated with painfully thin extremities, sunken eyes and concave cheeks; AIDS-associated seborrheic dermatitis crevassed his face with red, flaking patches—all hallmarks of advanced HIV infection.

I sat down next to him on the bed. "How're you feeling?" I asked. Despite my walking into the room with Louis, Allen was surprised to see me. Between coughing jags he reported "I'm okay. These Twix candy bars are really great. You should try them." He handed me a candy bar. I didn't need to ponder; I asked Louis to follow me into the kitchen. "Louis," I said, "we need to get him to a hospital. It looks bad." Having seen other manifestations of AIDS and cognizant of the never-ending midnight in which we lived, Louis was, sadly, not surprised. It was no great emergency, so we got into my car for the short drive to CPMC. One look at the diffusely, whited-out X-ray of his lungs confirmed that it was almost certainly *Pneumocystis*. We began treating his pneumonia immediately—although I had my suspicions that more was involved. A severe infection can affect mental capacity, of course, but Allen's cognition seemed more compromised than usual for a 45-year-old man with pneumonia. There was a three-day wait for MRIs, but I knew the radiology technicians well and they got him in for a head MRI the afternoon of my request. It showed multiple sites of pathology consistent with *Toxoplasmosis*— an infectious disease in the immunocompromised and often deadly for those with AIDS. We started him on antibiotics and Allen fully recovered from his PCP, but his brain *Toxoplasmosis* proved less easy to control and he never regained full mental capacity.

Because Allen and Louis owned their house on Scott Street with another business partner, Louis and the other investor bought out Allen's share of the house so they would not be stuck in a partnership with Allen's biologic family after Allen died, fearing that the family might want to sell the house to cash out. Allen's relationship with Louis, and the extraordinary attention which Louis provided during his last months, was nevertheless understood and appreciated by Allen's family. In fact Allen's mother and Louis maintained a relationship until she died in 2012. This was unlike many, many other families who appeared oblivious to the vigilant care provided by the partner of their son, brother or father. However, like the vast majority of families, Allen's was unwilling, or unable, to disclose the true cause of his death. Perhaps more families would have been able to discuss these diagnoses if our government had at least been willing to say the name: "AIDS." Instead, Allen's mother told her people that he had died of a brain tumor. Allen was hospitalized twice more in those six months before he stepped off the earth. That August we lost yet another friend.

LEARNING NOT TO ASK

During my early years at Columbia University in New York, I had struck up a friendship with Bill Kellerman, a smart, well-educated stockbroker who lived in San Francisco. Years after I met him, I was to see him again in California.

Bill had a two-bedroom apartment near the Castro. It was sometime in the late 1980s that he offered to rent his extra bedroom to a young man named Rick who had hit a rough time in finances. He had reason to step into Rick's room one day and he noticed a stack of lined paper which was so uniform that Bill initially thought it was fresh from a stationary store. On top of this stack, he found in a neat, cursive script a page with the sentence "I am a good person. I won't get AIDS." The sentence was repeated all the way down the page and covered each subsequent page all the way down to the bottom of the stack. This, it seemed to me, was a testament to the terror, confusion and magical thinking of the time.

When science is helpless, and the disease is as lethal as AIDS, it is no wonder that some people embraced their atavistic impulses and turned toward amulets and incantations, shamans and witch doctors.

Rick moved out of Bill's apartment and I didn't hear of him for a year and a half. When he eventually came to mind and I inquired about him, Bill said he'd heard Rick had committed suicide a few months earlier. It was this kind of answer, repeated over and over, which led me to stop asking about people. And so (after my Jack's death) I cultivated a fortress mentality: I stopped answering the phone, listening to phone messages and opening mail. I would tell myself that I would open the mail later, in a day or two, and

ANDREW M. FAULK, M.D.

it would stack, there on my living room coffee table, until the pile would become too unruly and spill over onto the floor. Eventually I would gather my strength, prepare for another death and open all the potential bomblets at once. But my system—if you can call it that—frequently failed and an envelope would go missing only to be found months later or not at all. To this day I find myself unable to immediately open unidentified mail or voice-mail when I suspect emotional content—I tell myself I'll open it when I'm feeling stronger... and prepared.

THE CHARM OF JACK'S WORLD

I met John Robert Soehlke, Jack to everyone, in the summer of 1987. I was preparing for the Board exam in Internal Medicine, but had gone out one night to the Eagle bar in San Francisco. (It seems most cities have a gay bar named the Eagle; if you want to find a gay bar in an unknown city, just look for a bar named the Eagle.)

Jack was a remarkable person with a staggering sense of comedy that, more often than not, took the form of physical humor. He stood about 5'8" with a small frame and an oversized grin. It was a ready smile, but not an "easy" one as there was effort in his enthusiasm which was, nonetheless, quick and undiluted. His skin had that tawny southern European hue but his last name, Soehlke, belied the Italian heritage he claimed—although, of course, surnames and ancestry ran more parallel a hundred years ago than they do today. He walked quickly, but with many extra steps as he backtracked and re-checked whatever task took up his attention in the moment. In less formal settings, his speech was punctuated by the squeals and tonal rises at the end of sentences normally associated with the hypothetical questions of old-fashioned "school marms" and some of our more flamboyant brothers—or as poking fun at both. His comic instincts were accurate but he was perfectly aware of the emotional temperature of his surroundings.

Jack was one of the few people I have known who was capable of joy, not just happiness, but joy. With that quality came an ambition and ability to inspire it among those around him. He didn't have the intellectual underpinnings to be especially witty with words or ideas for his humor was of a physical kind like that of Charlie Chaplin or Groucho Marx. He reproduced personality quirks and physical mannerisms of those around him with both hilarity and warmth. As with the great comedians, he would take a physical feature, usually kinetic, and reproduce it in an exaggerated, wonderfully entertaining, fashion. Much to the consternation of those around him unused to his ways, Jack would walk pretend stairs, tussle with imaginary crates and fight with unknown assailants. He would fall, convincingly, from unseen walls and mysterious precipices. He would struggle with mythical gates and argue with fabricated people. Sending museum guards into apoplexy, he would feign scratching a flake of paint off a priceless piece of art. He found his own performances delightful; I was charmed by their authenticity and audacity.

Jack used his voice as a major tool for his humor and it went from a high-pitched giggle to deep and dramatic hyper-masculine speech. His imagination was not constrained by social norms, and having an exceptionally malleable face, he could instantly turn a sympathetic or blank look into a mask of unbounded disbelief, unbridled sadness or faux horror. I have never seen anyone, excepting professional actors, so able to produce the quivering chin and trembling lips of impending tears. Groucho Marx had nothing on Jack when it came to listening in deep sincerity to someone and then turning away from his "target" to express either total disbelief or pure revulsion. He didn't keep it a secret from those who knew him when he was listening to something absurd from a speaker out of his depth or out of his mind. Because of his sense of humor, his mother judged him trivial and unmanly. I knew better.

But Jack had another quieter, supportive side characterized by an attentive focus on others. Just as he wanted to entertain others, he wanted to care for others, and perhaps that's really the same thing. He treated others, and certainly me, with thoughtfulness and generosity. For years after Jack's death, my parents, who had visited us in spite of some lingering qualms about my spiritual positioning, repeatedly remarked on his shouldering my care. I especially remember how it was after we moved to Los Angeles. It's difficult for me to explain my physical and mental state when I arrived home from work those days in Los Angeles. Jack would retrieve a soda from the refrigerator and say little but "hello." I would climb the stairs, then, of our two-story condo, shut the door to my study, and sit for awhile in complete silence to decompress from the emotional concussions of the day— the discouraging defeats, the never-ending explanations, the inspiring courage, the heart-breaking tragedies. Although managed as best I could, these matters were not, could not, be resolved in a few hours or days, months or even years. There were too many patients to see, tests to review and hospital visits to make to grieve every loss. And I found my own HIV perforating my emotional walls, and distress for my patients trickling into that sanctum "where I lived." It was a time when I assumed emotional shut-down of some kind was the only option; compartmentalization, a way to detach, I believed, was imperative. It was the only way I thought I could do what I did.

After an hour or so of preparing myself for a night of refuge, I would come back downstairs and there would be Jack: cheerful, innocent of the day's burdens and ignorant of my precarious journey through emotional chaos. His lightness balanced my heaviness. Had I calmed one patient's titanic rage at the husband by whom she had been infected? Jack pretended he needed assistance to boil water. Had I broken the news to Richard Speakman that he was HIV-positive? Jack feared his risotto was something useful only to NASA.

Rarely did I ever tell him the details of my work. He loved me, but could not provide intellectual solace. Yet Jack's comic relief did worlds to knit my shattered emotions back together. No matter the steady drumbeat of approaching calamity—the perpetual, random loss of friends and patients—Jack had the talent to create a change in my reference point. His excitement was irrepressible as he welcomed me home for the trial run of his new little fountain in our tiny backyard. He was unsuccessfully "teaching" the puppy to heel by voice command alone. Whether he was the comedian or the devoted spouse, he scattered tranquility as though he were a farmer seeding his fields.

For some time I was irritated by his lack of a job, but I soon came to rely on his care and humor and my annoyance lifted. He was employed for a short time as a perfume "sprayer" at the entrance to a large department store in the local mall, and while it lasted I'd receive reports of celebrity spotting and shopper disagreements which were made all the more entertaining by Jack's delivery. And when that job became too boring and unfulfilling and he returned to full-time homemaking, I was still regaled by stories of Tina Turner's sister (who lived in our complex) and the eccentricities of our other neighbors, which also included a policeman and a dancer for an aging movie star. Jack always had some piece of diversion for me, and I began to count on him more and more. Despite my anxieties and eccentricities, he loved taking care of me. At work I dealt with the sick and the suffering, the desperate and the dying and at night he did his best to wash away my discouragement and exhaustion. His efforts found a ready audience in me and I came home every night with gratitude and, I pray now, with acknowledgment. He was a balance in our home for my heavy heart.

THE MARRIAGE RING

In October of 1989, Jack and I took a vacation to Germany, Austria and Italy and it was there in Venice that I bought his ring. But before that, before my birthday, we visited Salzburg. Jack's favorite movie was *The Sound of Music* and even at home he would sometimes break into its trademark "The hills are alive..." in an exaggerated, overly-dramatic falsetto which was hilarious to hear coming from a grown man. While in Salzburg we discovered there was a *Sound of Music* tour which included a distant look at the historical Von Trapp home and some sites made famous by the film. I was a little embarrassed to go on such a commercialized, saccharine-infused tour which ran counter to my natural reserve. But Jack was delighted that such a tour existed, and once this came to light, there was absolutely no doubt we would be taking it.

Once aboard *The Sound of Music* bus, by Jack's choice we sat in the very front seats. I discovered, to my chagrin, that the bus was principally peopled by older women. We were the youngest wayfarers and the only other male was someone we assumed to be a husband who appeared as disgruntled and mortified as I felt. I myself wasn't as disgruntled as mortified, but I reasoned this was all due to my unattractive proclivity for occasional pretentiousness and that the tour should be appreciated for what it was. Such enjoyment, however, took time for me to cultivate and in the meantime my feelings bordered on humiliation. Shortly after the bus pulled away from the tourist depot, I was horrified to hear coming in chorus from the seat next to me the opening words "The hills are alive..." I slowly sank into my seat to appear as small as possible. But to my surprise, as Jack continued to sing the soaring, iconic song of *The Sound of Music*,

ANDREW M. FAULK, M.D.

from the back of the bus I began to hear others join along. Soon, the entire bus was singing "I go to the hills, when my heart is lonely..." There was nothing I could do, I was captive and my resistance was melting. "To sing through the night, like a lark who is learning to pray," I warbled. At the conclusion, irrepressible Jack began to sing it again in case anyone had missed out on a chorus.

During that trip to Europe we found ourselves in Venice, without planning, on my birthday. Walking down one of the narrow streets, we stumbled upon a small jewelry store in which we found a simple zircon ring of deep yellow gold, more yellow, we were told, than the gold that is sold in the U.S. Much of Jack's charm rose from his instant enthusiasm for various people, places, and things, and he immediately fell in love with the ring. Jack was not a man frequently drawn to physical objects, which made gift-giving occasions difficult, but knowing that this would make him happy, the ring was a windfall for me. I had discovered something which would please him, and something that was a universal symbol of love and attachment. In 1989 marriage equality wasn't on the horizon, and domestic partnership legalities weren't even in our consciousness, so a ring was the closest we came to symbolized commitment. By way of diversion, however, I told him that I didn't think as much of the ring as he did and that we couldn't afford it anyway. We walked back to our hotel for a mid-afternoon nap and I could tell the ring was on his mind. On arriving the concierge handed the key to Jack, who promptly pretended to drop it. We searched but I knew the location of the room key was not the mystery it seemed. Jack spent several minutes looking around the floor, even bringing in innocently helpful, hapless strangers until he "discovered" it. The concierge, who seemed to quickly catch on, wasn't entertained—but I was.

Up in the room, I pretended to nap while Jack slipped outside. Once he was gone, I raced to the jewelry store and bought the gold ring. Hoping to reach the hotel before he could return, I ran along the narrow, confusing streets. But Jack and I both reached the entrance to the hotel at the same time and both pretended that running into each other was expected. As if supplementary excursions were part of our tour, neither of us attempted an explanation. In his hands he carried an Italian version of a birthday cake and in my back pocket I carried the gold ring. That night, at some Venetian restaurant, we presented each other with our gifts. One of my cherished memories is of Jack's response: his smile sparkled more than usual and lasted throughout dinner and the walk home. And in the morning it was as bright as the night before.

After returning to the States I had the zircon exchanged for a diamond. Jack was so pleased that eventually it took a jeweler's warning before he halted the repetitive polishing of the ring: the setting would disappear, after all, if polished to excess.

THE DIAGNOSIS THAT BROKE MY HEART

While Jack was without a full-time job when we met in San Francisco in 1987, he usually worked as a distributor of low-end perfumes and occasionally as a window dresser for various department stores. But I think the work he enjoyed the most was arranging flowers. We'd been dating for a number of months when he got a job arranging flowers for a friend's wedding in Los Gatos, which is about an hour south of the city. As usual in that deadly serious tone of his which was often followed by a high-pitched giggle, he reminded me about his technique for evaluating his various bouquets, "Now you have to squint your eyes and look at the entire arrangement to really appreciate the colors and pattern!" Turning toward his creations at the front of the church, by way of example he peered through lids squeezed nearly shut. Squinting your eyes and looking at the whole, I thought, was his philosophy of life—a philosophy I could deeply appreciate. After the wedding was over and the clean-up finished, we headed back to San Francisco with Jack driving my car while I napped in the passenger seat.

He had had a dry cough for the preceding three days. In that trip back to the city, I napped intermittently and when we arrived in San Francisco, we stayed in my apartment that night. At around 2 a.m. I was awakened by his coughing and shortly afterwards he began to develop "air hunger" which was ominous. I read his temperature which was a startling 102.5 and took out my stethoscope and listened to his lungs: my heart sank when I heard a bilateral ("double") pneumonia; he almost certainly had PCP. Although a pneumonia was frightening, usually it could be successfully treated, but the implication it conveyed was devastating—Jack was immunocompromised and he had AIDS.

He was dying and I felt I barely had had the chance to get to know him. And could I, was I prepared to, walk him down that path? I had seen enough to know the consequences of caring for someone who was dying of the disease. We had only been dating for a short time, and it would have been understandable had I ended our relationship then. I had previously told myself, considering what I had seen and knowing what I knew, that I wouldn't get involved with anyone facing end-stage HIV, since the stress involved would fuel the progression of my own virus. But he and I had clicked in a beautiful way and I never seriously considered breaking off the relationship.

As Jack didn't know, and didn't want to know, his HIV status, we had negotiated our relationship carefully. It was my policy to strongly encourage everyone to be tested, but I didn't pressure them as I knew learning one's status could be psychologically devastating, and I trusted individuals to know whether knowing was best for them. It was a trade-off. Careful attention to yourself could give early warning of opportunistic diseases, but constant stress could fuel HIV's flame. He had had a prior partner, Ted, who had been hyper-vigilant for any newly appearing signs of AIDS, especially Kaposi's Sarcoma, but his maniacal inspections had been pointless as he died from AIDS anyway, his stress probably accelerating his infection. Whether or not a patient agreed to the test, I vigorously pushed safe sex strategies like not having sex while high and faithfully using condoms placed in strategic locations, and even those unlikely places like a car's glove compartment or a kitchen cabinet. I could not have been more forceful in condemning the use of unsterilized needles. During those years having paranoia about one's health may have been largely pointless, but it wasn't unusual. We were, after all, in the Dark Ages.

In carrying out the logistics for Jack's hospitalization, I buried my emotions for I believed that my feelings had to be "postponed." As would happen time and again later in my medical career, emotionally dealing in the moment was an expenditure of time and energy I mistakenly believed I could ill afford. Now I understand that even in the worst of circumstances, even when emotional expression seems too overwhelming to be handled immediately, sorrow is best experienced at a time of loss; delay only inflicts a greater psychological price. But surprising as it may sound, at the age of 33 I was still a child when it came to coping with such feelings. I can't judge myself

ANDREW M. FAULK, M.D.

too harshly, though, for shutting down emotionally and postponing grief—it is a natural human reaction to choose a course which seems less painful in the moment, even when in the end it is more brutal. For a kernel of the grief was, of course, sorrow for my own losses: every relationship, every success, every passion, every dream was to be taken from me. Not in the distant future, not after 40 or 50 years, but soon. I had moved from a point in life where I was no longer experiencing the receiving years of youth, but the take-aways of an older age I had not yet attained.

I drove Jack to California Pacific where a friend in radiology agreed to do a chest X-ray off-record. As Jack waited in the radiology anteroom, I threw his chest film onto a light box and flipped it on. My heart sank—the film showed his lungs were whited out with the dense infiltrates of PCP. I felt as if I'd been socked in the stomach.

The experience of suddenly knowing my partner's diagnosis would be repeated 14 years later when (future partner) Lance Newman, in March 2002, was admitted to the University of California San Francisco hospital with chest pain. There, too, I saw the seriousness of his condition before he did. In the ER with Lance, I looked over the shoulder of the technician taking the 12-lead EKG and was shocked not only by the evidence of ongoing cardiac ischemia (oxygen deficiency), but also evidence of a "completed" heart attack sometime in the past. In both cases, I had the information before they did and my partners were far more ill than they knew. Occasionally, in a patient's mind, the physician is associated with the illness, and so it was best that I be on the patient's side of the diagnosis; in the doctor-patient equation, it was important that I stood with them and that they be informed by their own physician, not me. It fell to me to reassure them both, to reveal nothing by voice or facial expression, before their doctors told them their condition. I was a doctor, but I wasn't *their* doctor.

In case my examination of Jack at home, and the ubiquity of HIV, had not revealed the diagnosis, his chest X-ray did. He had received a death sentence and it was up to his physician to gauge how much of the information he should be told immediately, and how much to be given gradually. I said what I usually said and told him it looked like PCP, but that we needed more information for a final diagnosis.

As he didn't have medical insurance, I knew CPMC couldn't care for him and I would need to drive him to San Francisco General where those without insurance could receive care. Thankfully, I could step back.

We arrived at San Francisco General, and I stood by his side while he was admitted through the ER, a task made simpler and faster by the X-ray I held in my hands. He had a habit of "clucking" his tongue in a sound that communicated "this is the way it is—nothing can be done about it." It was to be a night filled with clucking. My emotions grew numb; a psychological distance between me and the information began to form. Although he took the diagnosis well, he knew what it meant. We didn't know how long he had; we didn't know how long any of us had. But in that uncertainty was a bit of hope. As we worked through admission and the beginning of treatment, his clucking intensified, but I saw quiet courage as I would see it in so many others and it is the response I hope to demonstrate when I approach my final days. I have never promised a particular response when it comes to my own final diagnosis—it may be yelling and screaming, hostility and rage. But, rather, I hope I'll have the calm bravery Jack had that night—the same courage I've seen in others over and over again.

The question was not if we were to die—we are all destined to die at some point. Rather it was when, the question was how soon. As if in battle, bombs were falling all around and we knew at any moment, without warning, we could be annihilated. Like those next to us, each day could be our last. Unlike a war zone, however, when our guys stepped off the earth, there was no loud explosion or cratered earth; our men went quietly to their graves. It seemed wrong for a life filled with talk and laughter, song and shouting, to end so early with only the quiet murmur of a faint exhale.

Had I been HIV-negative, who knows what my reaction would have been? Over the years I've contemplated again and again what my behavior would have been had I not been infected. Picturing such a state, I've always imagined that I would have locked myself in my career and in my apartment even more tightly than I had.

ANDREW M. FAULK, M.D.

NO HELP FROM THE PARENTS

Jack asked that I call his parents, Gus and Viv, and tell them he had a serious pneumonia. They lived in Collinsville, Illinois, a suburb of St. Louis, and this would be my first interaction with his parents. It did not go well. It quickly became apparent that his mother was more concerned about who had "given" him the disease than the details of his diagnosis and prognosis. As I was on the phone reporting his illness, I instantly became an easy target for her confusion and anger. I had given HIV to Jack, she concluded—for all intents and purposes, I had taken a gun and shot her son dead. Unfortunately that was to set the tone of our relationship as her grief morphed into anger. But her tone of voice, the words she chose, her overall reaction, wasn't entirely anger at me; Viv was also angry with Jack. His behavior had been irresponsible, she believed, and no matter the timing of HIV's discovery, he deserved his illness. It was a reaction I heard many times from many others who obviously didn't take into account that only one exposure by one person was all that was necessary for infection, just as one event is all that's needed for a pregnancy. Of course it was easy to condemn gay men with HIV, for their sexual activity itself, already the central preoccupation of the heterosexual world, was judged repugnant. Sometimes she communicated her disgust in words and sometimes just in her tone of voice. It was an ugly way of dealing with the disease and sometimes came from family members who had never accepted their son or brother's sexual orientation to begin with.

That first day in the hospital, when Jack was formally diagnosed with PCP, I was bending over him with my stethoscope listening to his heart, when he breathed a very audible wheeze. I showed no outward sign of hearing the abnormality. He, on the other hand, reacted to it: his face contorted not into a mask of heartbreak or horror, but rather into a facetious register of contrived alarm and sham distress. Imagine, not fear and despair, but faux devastation in a hospital room! But it was Jack's nature to bypass these reactions with a humor born from detached amusement and an optimism of unknown origin. Although there were many other reasons, I loved him for this.

I went home that night exhausted. I had slept little in the chair next to his bed the night before and I had to return to work the next day. In spite of his parents' judgmental response, they remained much of the week before flying back to Illinois. But I was correct in my immediate take that they would not be helping me handle Jack's condition. Viv, it seems, lived in a state of constant anger. She was angry long before his diagnosis and would remain so, I believed, long after he passed away. Her critical attitude was to show up repeatedly. Once, when I took them out to dinner in Collinsville, she deftly turned my victory into defeat when she complained about the salad and accused the restaurant of adding sugar. Later she announced to the restaurant at large that the smells emanating from the fish at the next table were making her nauseous. So it was a frosty reception I received when they first entered his hospital room that day. Jack's father, Gus, took most of his cues from Viv, but he nevertheless treated Jack with a compassion that Viv's anger would not allow. Being a retired high school gym instructor, he coached Jack with the tools he had, suggesting that physical exercises would speed up healing. Gus gave what he could and performed examples of his exercises. Although his naïveté may have been painful to watch, his loving contribution was deeply moving. Jack, however, clucked his tongue so often that week that even he noticed it, but it was a compulsion he could not control.

In spite of my own opinion of the emotional state of his parents, I realized that, for my sake, things would go better if I allowed them some forgiveness. He was their son, after all, and they were as upset and afraid as I was.

After recovering from his bout with PCP, Jack did remarkably well on *Pneumocystis* prophylaxis and the heavy, usually debilitating, doses of AZT prescribed at the time. His energy and outlook remained at their usual high. Approaching death was on his mind,

ANDREW M. FAULK, M.D.

of course, but he rarely discussed this, nor allowed fear or self-pity to overwhelm him. He knew, however—we both knew—that his final illness was inevitable and, in all probability, soon. We were wrong, as he was not diagnosed with HIV-related Non-Hodgkin's Lymphoma until late 1990 and lived until 1991.

STARTING A PRACTICE

After graduating from my Internal Medicine Residency at CPMC in 1987, I was the only one of my class to be asked to join an established medical practice in town. In the end this was to prove a mixed blessing. I was to take the place of Wayne Bayless, M.D., a retiring doctor in Dr. Jim Carlton's office, which, because of the additional manpower my association would produce, would formally link up with Dr. John Lore's practice. Dr. Bayless had a practice largely made up of bread-and-butter general practice patients. This demographic was similar to John Lore's practice. James Carlton had, on the other hand, a growing HIV practice. Both physicians were gay and I was ecstatically relieved to finally come out in my profession. Because of the potential legal ramifications, however, my HIV status was to remain a secret, even from my eventual colleagues at Lawrence Medical in L.A. But, for the first time, I no longer needed to hide my sexual orientation.

John Lore was the more down-to-earth, nuts-and-bolts, entrepreneurially savvy of the two docs. Jim Carlton, on the other hand, was the classic image of the absent-minded professor: it even showed in his tentative gait which would stop-and-start as he talked and then thought. Jim would appear to be physically lost even when he wasn't. John Lore, on the other hand, was as sophisticated and polished as Jim Carlton was not—John laughed easily and knew exactly what to say to put patients and their families at ease and inspire trust, but though Carlton and Lore were an unlikely pair, they were equal in the quality of care they delivered to their patients. Each was an academic and consistently up-to-date in his knowledge of diagnoses and treatments. My newly forming practice was anticipated to be two-thirds HIV patients, the overflow of Dr. Carlton's practice, and one-third the overflow of Dr. Lore's practice. Dr. Lore's practice, it turned out, was an amalgam of older people, principally women, and rising young professionals of both genders. With our new association, John Lore moved his office space next door to Jim Carlton's. There was much discussion as to how to combine the two disparate populations—the majority being young men, who had a real possibility of being clearly HIV patients (perhaps emaciated, coughing, and with visible KS lesions), and the minority being the mixture of elderly women and up-and-coming professionals. We thought carefully of how to preserve both types of practices. John Lore's moving his practice next door to Jim Carlton's allowed me to have access to both waiting rooms: John Lore's reserved for the non-HIV patients and Jim Carlton's for the growing HIV population. Two separate waiting rooms seemed the best way to make both groups comfortable.

THE HOSTILE RECEPTIONIST

Unfortunately for my career in San Francisco, my relationship with their receptionist, Dorothy, had quickly soured after my practice began. Dorothy, dressed in a nurse's uniform complete with white cardboard tiara, but with no more than a high school education, made my days with Carlton and Lore an embarrassment that blossomed into a nightmare. From my office I could hear her on the phone giving patients badly flawed recommendations which were distressingly dangerous. Once during a pelvic exam, with my patient full in the table stirrups, Dorothy had interrupted by banging on the door and loudly insisting I come out immediately to attend to a hospitalized patient. Dorothy constantly spoke to me as if she were the responsible physician and I was the untutored receptionist. In fact Dorothy spoke to both Carlton and me as if we were delinquent children. To see my patients' reactions to her condescending abuse was not only distressing but fraught with potential consequence: if the receptionist-secretary needed to "manage" me this way, could patients be expected to trust me?

As I had purchased the part of the practice that belonged to Dr. Wayne Bayless, I was gradually paying him slowly decreasing percentages of my earnings. After my payments to Bayless, however, I was barely making more than my expensive parking bills in the downtown San Francisco building which housed our offices. As my schedule in the Carlton/Lore office was constantly full, rough calculations of what my pay should have been was beginning to make me wonder if Dorothy was practicing some creative bookkeeping— doctor offices were famous for staff embezzlement. As if to prove my point, two years after I left the practice the IRS knocked on my door with not one but two errant "W-2s." Evidently she had been generously helping herself to the office till while attributing her extra income to me and sticking me with the taxes on it, which I dutifully paid.

Throughout my career I've tried to keep my patient's appointments and have them wait as little as possible—this is, obviously, the goal of every physician. But sometimes patients are double-booked to prevent any unproductive "down time." This was not my particular style and I informed Dorothy of this fact. Nevertheless she overbooked me repeatedly. When I called her on her objectionable scheduling, she said that this was Dr. Bayless' routine way of doing things. And then she would return to whatever she was doing to let me know that the conversation was over. (My most enduring image of Dorothy is of her sitting at her desk studiously painting over her mistakes with "White Out.")

My attempt to demand office changes went badly, but was as disturbingly fascinating as a car crash. Out of the office, on the tiny back deck of my small apartment, I told Jim Carlton of my problems with Dorothy. Jim Carlton's response was not only dismissive but also revealed unwanted Freudian insight into his curious mentality. He responded to my complaints, "Oh, if you think she's hard to live with, you should have been around my mother." I was astonished! His extraordinarily inappropriate response was outrageous on so many levels. It was an indication of my naïveté that when I finally presented my suspicions of her financial infidelity, and consequently presented Jim with the ultimatum that either she or I leave the office, he took not a heartbeat to thank me for my time working in their office.

Parenthetically, in spite of the indignity of his instant choice of the madwoman Dorothy, I will always have a soft spot for the painfully insecure and voluntarily-abused Jim Carlton. Often when I phoned Jim's home, I would hear another man's voice on his answering machine. Upon questioning John Lore about this, he told me that it was the voice of Jim's partner who had died long ago—it was a recording Jim couldn't bring himself to substitute with his own message. This was not unusual: across the city telephones were being answered with the voices of long-passed lovers. The day before Jack died, I myself recorded a new greeting over the endearingly playful message Jack had recorded—I knew once he was gone I'd never have the strength to erase the message I'd come to know intimately and love dearly.

A LOOK BACK AT THE PROFESSIONAL CLOSET

Throughout my residency and internship at CPMC, there were, as there always are, references in records and people's remarks about other doctors, former doctors. On questioning I would hear the names and short stories of other gay M.D.s who had died from AIDS. As was routine back in those days, you learned of others' passing in short asides.

"Oh, this doc, I don't see him caring for so-and-so anymore."

"Yes, he passed away last year."

"Really? How old was he?" (Don't we always question the ages of the deceased to compare ourselves to those who have passed? If they're younger, or just plain young, we press to know details. Could we be subject to a similar twist of fate?)

"I don't know, early thirties I'd guess. He died of AIDS."

The longer I was at CPMC, the more I felt the ghosts of these former physicians.

Certainly my years in pre-med classes left me with an abiding sense of vulnerability and, though the ridiculous tie-cutting imbroglio with Dr. LeFou at the UW had nothing to do with my sexual orientation, it reinforced a sense of easy replacement and casual substitution.

I had come out to myself and to close friends, but the professional world was quite a different matter. I resolved the conundrum by forming my own internal code: I wouldn't come out professionally until I had every diploma, every license, that I could possibly want. If I hadn't had such a fixed policy, the judgments and decision-making would have been constant. However necessary they were, I still occasionally have feelings of embarrassment about these deceptions.

My carefully thought out strategy of concealment owing to my professional vulnerability was fast becoming unnecessary, and it was time for a reassessment of those earlier maneuvers. I anticipated the day when I could leave this policy behind.

After I'd finished the residency requirements for Board Certification in Internal Medicine, the necessary examination followed. In order to prepare, I signed up for a one week Internal Medicine review class in San Diego. In classrooms people often sit in the same seats, day after day, and I was no exception; each day found me close to the front. During the course, there were multiple occasions when the reviewer asked a question, and the audience was given the chance to answer. I found myself comparing whispered answers with a nattily dressed physician sitting next to me. I happened to answer many of these questions correctly—the gentleman sitting next to me, not as frequently. As the week progressed, I began to eat lunch with him and we exchanged our personal stories. Vincent Briar, M.D. had taken the exam several times already, and had yet to pass. He was in practice with Fred Lawrence, M.D. in Los Angeles; together they formed a partnership, Lawrence Medical Group, which was made up of several physicians, doctor assistants and a psychologist.

On Thursday of this week-long review, at lunch Vincent Briar, M.D. asked me if I were gay. My work in the Lore/Carlton office had not yet begun and my historic policy remained in place: no professional disclosure until I passed the Medical Board exam. I told him no, I wasn't gay.

"Although I'm straight, I work in a gay practice with primarily gay patients. For us, sexual orientation is not an issue," Vincent informed me.

That night I went back to the hotel and pondered what I had said. I debated with myself throughout the evening—Vincent's question, of course, had been an innocent one. The winds of change were blowing across the country and I was just one exam away from Board Certification. All the intense years of medical school, internship and residency were behind me. I realized that I was no longer professionally vulnerable; whatever this stranger from L.A. thought of me would not impact my final goal. The next day, Friday, was the last day of the course and at lunch I sheepishly told Vincent I was gay. I explained my reasoning and standing policy, although no explanation was needed for Vincent—he understood perfectly. He

ANDREW M. FAULK, M.D.

immediately offered me a position at Lawrence Medical which I declined; I already had a job with the newly-combined practice of John Lore and Jim Carlton. He told me to keep his offer in mind, however, and we exchanged business cards.

Although I'd had a logical and understandable policy in place, it was time for it to be discarded, time for me to come out of my carefully constructed closet. It took some courage to identify myself fully to Dr. Briar, but the redemption made it worthwhile and was a taste of the professional freedoms to come.

It was months later, when I had been driven nearly insane by Dorothy's monarchy, that I resigned—disregarding the common sense rule that one should never abandon a job without another in hand. It was precisely the last day of my tenure at the Dr. Carlton/ Mother Dorothy circus that I got Vincent's call from L.A. He had an HIV patient relocating to San Francisco—could I follow him?

"No, Vincent, I can't help you," I said, "I won't be in practice here anymore." I summarized Dorothy's imperial behavior and Jim's response to my naïve "her or me" ultimatum.

Once again, Vincent Briar offered me a job on the spot.

FRED LAWRENCE, M.D.

I had initially refused Vincent Briar's early offers to join Lawrence Medical in Los Angeles; my wounds were still fresh from the Lore/Carlton debacle. How could I be sure I wasn't walking into another office with behavioral and ethical problems? Besides, I didn't want to leave a city that had made itself a unique home for gay people, Bohemians, and misfits, a haven of political and sexual tolerance. San Francisco had been my first exposure to California and I was hypnotized by the foggy weather and surrounding natural beauty. (This was before the turn of the last century after which it became significantly larger and substantially different.) I saw L.A., on the other hand, as its famous cliché—a sweltering, intellectual wasteland consumed by superficial appearance and political apathy. Mistaking my snobbery and suspicion for strategy, Briar offered more incentive: he suggested a trial run. For working in L.A. one week a month, the practice would pay me the equivalent of a month's work in San Francisco plus airfare to Los Angeles and back. It was a plan that won me over; soon I was flying back and forth in order to work one week a month in the LMG office. Instead of General Dorothy, I discovered Rhonda, their chief receptionist. She was efficient, playful and had that sixth sense of knowing which situations required immediate attention. Their office was not only friendly and harmonious, but also well-run. It took only a few months of such courtship to win me over, and soon Jack and I were temporarily living in a small hotel in Hollywood.

It was appropriate that Fred Lawrence lived in the spotlight for he was larger than life. He was a force of nature who had achieved wealth and prestige by seizing opportunities that others either didn't see or didn't have the audacity to exploit. He thought large. The Roman philosopher Seneca said that luck is what happens when preparation meets opportunity. If that is so, Fred had done a lot of preparing and when it came to opportunities, Fred had usually created them too. With his imagination and abilities, he could transform a bad undertaking into a good one and, if that was not possible, discard it with speed and finesse. Fred saw expansion where others saw risk, bargains where others saw junk, and the gifted and the capable where others saw the ordinary and the troublesome.

Sometime during the 1970s he had been a *Playgirl* centerfold. At the time, he had such compelling good looks that the magazine had placed him front and center, literally. Oddly enough, I had seen that particular issue in the '70s, though later than its printing, lying about in the not-fit-for-renting apartment that my friend Norman Nash kept as his New York *pied-à-terre* on West 19th Street. But I saw the issue again during the course of my work at Lawrence Medical Group when Fred himself showed it to me. It was not that he left it lying about for the world to see. He had brought it into the office and, protecting it from any uninvited glance, showed it to me alone. Had I myself ever looked that becoming and received such exposure, I suspect the walls of my office, including waiting room and patients' bathroom, would have been wallpapered with the issue.

Lawrence had been one of the very first doctors to advertise. His ads often took whole pages of the local gay rag and, later, smaller portions of national magazines. He occasionally placed photos of the other docs in these ads, so my face and specialized area of practice became somewhat recognizable in the community. As I was becoming known as an HIV physician, greeting a patient in the street might be an indication of someone's positive HIV status and so I never acknowledged a patient first. Without their greeting I behaved as if I'd never seen them. Not everyone understood this tactic, and it led some to conclude I was cold and aloof.

One of Fred's maxims was "punctuality is power" and that if one wished for a particular item or study, one had to be sitting at the table on time. After learning this, I was often early at morning meetings and became privy to remarks not necessarily intended for staff or peers. Despite his career, he drove his Mercedes-Benz with the speed and abandon of a NASCAR 500 racer—clearly he liked to nurture a bad-boy image. Pam was his personal assistant as well as the glue holding together the diverse subdivisions of our practice. It was at several morning meetings that I heard Pam and him discuss his latest speeding ticket and the various penalties—such as traffic school—that he would be forced to endure.

Vincent rather than Fred had recruited me, so I first met Fred while he was house hunting in the Hollywood Hills. While he found me acceptable, the house he was examining that day was not. In only a matter of months, though, I was integrated into the efficient, happy staff of Lawrence Medical and Fred had found a quirky house on Outpost Drive which was complete with a small waterfall, holding pond, swimming pool and changing cabana.

At the LMG office, staff called Fred Lawrence "doctor" as if the word "doctor" were a name itself. I thought this system was a brilliant invention. The custom couldn't extend to us, however—we were always called "Dr. so-and-so." After all, it would be confusing to have more than one physician in the office called simply "doctor." It's similar to parenting, this situation of benign authority: parents should not necessarily be friends with their children. Although there are exceptions with long-term friends in a physician's office, it's usually not helpful to morph a relationship into what technically it is not. Especially in these situations in which we were dealing with life and death, people need to view their physician as that and little else.

Fred was a "quality" dresser, with designer suits that fit him flatteringly. He ate at fine restaurants almost exclusively with an entourage of two to five who orbited around him like so many planets around a star. In my time this included his interior decorator, a Frenchman, Jacques Charmant, who seemed to live with him on and off. In fact, for my parents' first visit to my new office in Los Angeles, we had met Fred in a trendy restaurant with his constellation of subjects in full gravitational pull. In an over-the-top remark consistent with his style, he thanked my parents for birthing me, as I was "a gift to medicine" and certainly to his humble practice. Jacques kissed my mother's outstretched hand upon being introduced which was perfectly in keeping with Fred's sense of style and ceremony and which surprised and charmed her.

LAWRENCE MEDICAL GROUP—
AN EARLY, AND FAVORITE, PATIENT

In one of my first weeks in L.A., I saw patient Chris Carley. Lawrence Medical had one custom that was incredibly helpful for patient care. Upon first being seen by the practice, the patient was photographed there at the front desk with a resulting instant photo. It was a terrific idea, giving doctors and staff an easy memory aid for telephone calls or M.D. "sign-offs" for night or week-end coverage. I recall his entering photo—Chris, blond, blue-eyed, looking young and robust at 30 and yet uncomfortable under the lens of the camera.

I'm not sure why I took a special interest in him—perhaps it was his quiet, introverted way or maybe his unassuming personality resonated with my own. As was the norm he had come in for his initial HIV results alone but as I got to know him he seemed socially isolated. Besides encouraging group therapy, Fred often recommended patients invest in a large TV. Frequently, as the disease progressed, watching TV became a patient's only entertainment and too often their only friend. For whatever reasons, perhaps partially due to the stigma of sexual orientation, many patients were without close friends or family which left them alone and lonely in darkened bedrooms with a TV their only company.

Chris asked for me on his return appointments and complained of very little during his office visits; his being seen was almost always for follow-up to monitor his health and determine if any new medication had been discovered to treat HIV. He seemed slightly more fearful than most patients I saw, but he carried it in a quiet way, without histrionics or morbid speculation. It was obvious he didn't enjoy being in an exam room, but he shouldered this discomfort in a workman-like way. Chris, like most patients in the practice, was usually seen alone and, despite the discomfort he felt being examined and discussing his illness, he seemed content in his solitude. That comfort in solitude seemed the most compelling characteristic he and I had in common.

As Chris's T-cells slipped lower and lower, it seemed to me that his isolation was more and more of an impediment and that his life would be prolonged, and happier, if there was someone providing some support. And as for my universal advice to "Get happy!" he seemed unable to do that. I sensed that others could provide a happiness, and of course support, that his routine solitude could not.

As his health deteriorated, I delved deeper into his social support. He had a mother living somewhere in the San Joaquin Valley of California but no father and no siblings; he seemed to have few, if any, friends. As the horizon of his life inched into view, I pushed him harder and harder to tell his mother, if no one else, of his HIV diagnosis. He resisted and I should probably have seen that as evidence of a parent who was unable to help her son in any crisis. I was to discover in hindsight that involving his mother in his care was hardly the best answer for Chris's life.

During one of our discussions, it seemed apparent that he was working out the end of his life alone. I pressed him to inform his mother. I said I would be happy to discuss the situation with her, in his presence, if he felt that might be helpful. He overcame his intuitive reluctance, finally, and came in with his mother. As they entered my exam room, he told me, under his breath, that he had disclosed his positive status to her just that morning. As I explained the medical situation and the unknown variables in his condition, she increasingly demonstrated a disturbing narcissism. Her questions revolved around herself and her own reaction to his illness, not to him or his ordeals. There, in front of him, she voiced her fears of what his illness would do to her and of how his sexuality and disease made it impossible for her to inform those in her own social support network. When she began questioning infectivity and her own safety in being around her son, his eyes glazed over. Clearly, I had made a mistake in pushing him to bring his mother into the loop.

In January of 1991, my world was crumbling around me—by then, Fred Lawrence was ill and Jack was undergoing chemotherapy at the University of California Los Angeles (UCLA) hospital. Chris's downward spiral was another blow, albeit lesser, to my psychological equilibrium. The last time I saw him alive he was hospitalized in a large room at the Medical Center of North Hollywood. Although the sun had set, the shades were drawn. The TV was off and his hospital tray stand stood with nothing on it except a styrofoam cup with a straw in it. The back of his bed was raised and there, silhouetted by the fluorescent light panel behind him, Chris sat in a space empty of sound and people and stared ahead into a vacant room and the desolate future before him.

He was bright enough to know medicine had little to offer beyond pain control, indeed he asked no questions about further treatment. Words failed in the tableau before me; offering hope to this man would have been an affront to his intelligence. My efforts to create a social structure to combat his isolation hadn't worked—the meeting with his mother had been a miserable failure. Despite opiates for his pain, he lay awake, mentally intact and aware of approaching death. In our last days, most of us fear pain and loss of personal autonomy, but he had control of his bodily functions, so I asked him whether or not he was in pain. He replied no, but said nothing more. I couldn't read anything in his face and although I'm comfortable with silence, the quiet here was agonizing. I was walking into a familiar situation yet it was unfamiliar at the same time. Often distant patients became surprisingly accessible when they're confronted with approaching death, but this was not to be Chris Carley's way. I began to see, however, that I didn't have to say anything profound. I could give him quite possibly the most important gift any of us can give the dying—our presence.

In those days, before the advent of laptop computers and digitized patient records, physicians would sit at the centralized nursing desks and write out in longhand reports of patients' progress and orders for tests and therapies. Nurses disliked any removal of patients' charts from their stations because their absence could be a source of escalating confusion. I understood: I appreciated the need for a central location for information. But my connectedness with those in my care was paramount, and I felt it could best be obtained by charting in Chris' room. I gathered all the records of my various patients and moved them into his room, sat down in a chair next to his bed, and began the process of charting. I believe that my quiet presence next to my guys provided what routine medical training and expertise could not.

When I charted in the hospital, I often would choose the patient who was the most ill or isolated and work in his room, next to his bed. Sometimes these patients were barely conscious, sometimes they were awake and talkative. Whether it was due to social abrasiveness, or perhaps conspicuous eccentricities, there were always some of my patients who had few social skills and fewer friends; it was not unusual for many to face their illness more or less alone. Although I needed quiet in which to write my notes and orders, this was usually an hour or so in which I could be a presence for my patients.

GEORGE KRIVACEK AND LLOYD BURR

It was during my first days in the HIV clinic Fred Lawrence had lovingly engineered that I was introduced to George Krivacek, a long-standing patient. He was an immigrant from what was then Czechoslovakia and his occupation was buying houses, restoring or improving them, and then reselling them. George had the aristocratic manners of old Europe and the financial know-how of the flintiest businessman. He and his partner, Lloyd Burr, lived in the Hollywood Hills.

Besides being a patient, George and his partner Lloyd soon became good friends, with Jack and me dining at their house on several occasions. When Jack and I moved to Valley Village, George had loaned me money to help buy our condo. My midwestern values were such that I borrowed from no one other than the bank and George. (It was only later I learned that hefty down payments on California real estate were misguided where the value of one's property could easily zero out with fire or earthquakes, as mine did after the Northridge earthquake of 1994.) In any case, one of the most haunting memories I have is that of sitting down to dinner at George and Lloyd's, with Jack and me on one side of the table, George and Lloyd across from us, eating a simple dinner. I tried, even then, to freeze such images in my mind, as I was acutely aware we were all living on borrowed time and that such pleasant events could not last. We were, after all, the children of Hamelin and my sense of foreboding was all too accurate. Of the group, Jack would be the first to die. Later, Lloyd's alcoholism led to his own violent death in that very dining room and George, the last of the three, wouldn't survive the ravages of "Compound Q." And yet there stands that image of our group enjoying the simplest of pleasures and camaraderie—making a simple salad, sitting down together for dinner—as if we were protected from the hurricane crashing around us and had all the time in the world. It's a memory that comes back to me time and again for I'm successful in preserving those images, but am painfully aware that I'm the only one left to recall them.

ANDREW M. FAULK, M.D.

TRUST AND RESPECT

Early on at LMG, on the chart placed on the door of the examination room, I found a female patient's name. Placing the patient's chart outside the exam room is a foundation of clinical practice for obvious reasons and is unlikely to change. In any case I found this chart without the routine Polaroid photo attachment. According to her file, she appeared very healthy and was HIV-negative. Half prepared, I adjusted myself for a new patient, at least new to me.

She was Fred Lawrence's ex-wife in for her annual physical. At first I wondered why she was in our practice; then I puzzled over why she was given to me. "Whatever," I told myself, as I provided her with one of the best exams I've ever performed. The write-up afterwards was similarly one of the better ones of my career. (I've read the post-mortem of President John F. Kennedy after his assassination and I've wondered why it was done by what seemed a first-year medical student.) Although one is never to treat their own family, I never asked why Fred had given a VIP patient to me in particular.

As my time at LMG progressed, I also did exams of Fred's mother who was our Chief Financial Officer, as well as Fred's brother and his nephew. I understood the responsibility for these exams was a testament to Fred's faith in me.

THE WORST MOMENT, READY OR NOT

Diagnosis—the very worst moment of someone's life. Like my own experience in San Francisco, the office employed the only reasonable policy: we never gave results, positive or negative, over the telephone for we wanted one of our physicians or our psychologist present. Without this understanding clearly stated in advance, asking someone to come in for an office visit would have telegraphed their status. Once in the office, I would convey the report in a supportive manner. I had to transmit a certainty about the finding, but also that ingredient which keeps all of us alive—hope.

Before breaking the news, I would take a minute in the hallway to still myself—to separate from whatever I had been dealing with before. After having told the staff that I could not take calls, I would walk into the room and sit down. When a physician stands, it gives a message that he is in a hurry and on his way out; it gives the impression that the patient doesn't have his undivided attention or, worse, that the issue at hand is inconsequential. Whoever was receiving this information deserved his doctor's full attention and eye-to-eye intimacy. There would be no beating around the bush or drama as I would tell the patient immediately in no uncertain terms. There could be no confusion that either the test had been performed incorrectly or that the result might be that of someone else. I'd answer their questions of "Are you sure this is my test? Are you sure it's positive?" There was no mistake here: the results were what they were and without a doubt applied to the person sitting in front of me. After the certainty of the test results, I'd present the uncertainty of prognosis—which was, after all, a piece of hope. I would give them the truth about epidemics in general. Carefully avoiding the word "survive" and instead favoring the softer expression "do well," I'd say yes, this was a bad finding, but in every epidemic throughout history there were those who did well. In HIV we didn't know who these people were, but that was cause for hope! How were we to know that any one person wasn't in that group that did well? I gave out no estimates, however, of any one particular person's lifespan—my non-scientific gross observations of a 10% long-term survival rate were unproven and, of course, unpublished. It was not for me to blindly guess someone's chances of survival.

Every time I would give a little hope, a voice would whisper in my ear: "but not for you." The odds for any of us weren't good; even should the long-term survival rate be 30%, the mortality rate would still stand at a catastrophic 70%.

So I believed I was not to survive this virus. And, odds were, neither were my patients. So it was with much surprise that I gradually came to realize that I was one of those fortunate few who were to survive years—if not many years. It was bittersweet irony when it became clear that I would live to see most of my patients die.

GIVING THE NEWS

Besides giving out the HIV result, there were the hard times of telling someone just how serious HIV was. So much depended on the individual. How ready were they to hear such news? How sick were they at that moment sitting in front of me? Were they psychologically strong enough to be told immediately they were to die soon? This judgment, the right call, was just as much a part of my practice as ordering tests and writing prescriptions.

One might assume that anyone knowing he had HIV would know it was lethal. Yes, some were ready; they had surmised what a blood test or a ratifying CT or X-ray would confirm. Others were in such denial that even ongoing symptoms didn't penetrate their conscious awareness. It was my duty, my solemn work, to map this terrain of the soul and convey the seriousness of the situation while leaving room for hope. As part of this strategy, I wouldn't answer questions which weren't asked; I would wait for the patient to lead me to their hopes and fears. I wouldn't rush. I would take my time.

As my own physician, Mark Higgins, M.D., remarked to me years later, a person's all-important expectations depended on how many people with AIDS he knew, because this experience provided insight words couldn't. Many patients who had watched their counts drift lower and lower knew others who had preceded them and were ready. I won't ever forget those who had the gallows humor to joke about naming their few remaining T-cells. I found that those who were most ready for the worst news, not surprisingly, were those who had begun experiencing that long list of "take-aways" that HIV demanded—those who had lost their friends and faculties, their capabilities and independence, those who had had illness after illness until the disease simply wore them out. There were those who had been scorched by the fire and were ready to step off the earth.

* * *

One of the most memorable patients was a man in his early thirties who presented in the office without having had previous medical care. Although he'd lost 30 lbs. he was still remarkably handsome. Light blue eyes with jet black hair, perhaps "Black Irish," he worked in one of the majority of jobs that are respectable but without high profile. Besides the obvious weight loss, his face was marked by the telling seborrheic dermatitis with its heavy flaking and redness at the edges of his nose and the space between his eyebrows. In his case, the staff had taken one look at him, listened to his complaints and sent him for a chest X-ray even before I had seen him.

He was in denial about the extent of his illness. I did a quick exam, listened to his lungs and then took his film into the hall where our light box was located. His chest X-ray was a snow storm of *Pneumocystis*. I walked back into the exam room and told him it looked like a bad pneumonia. Blood had yet to be drawn, and so I didn't have the hard data of his HIV test. I looked into his eyes and judged his readiness to receive the horrendous news: not only did he almost certainly have PCP, but the length of his life was probably going to be measured in days, maybe weeks, but certainly not months. I told him the pneumonia looked bad and that he'd need to be admitted to the hospital, but I didn't say he had PCP or AIDS. In his early thirties and not having had a sick day in his life, in the way he presented himself, I felt he wasn't ready to be told he was dying. He needed some time to digest, to let others take care of him and allow some of the overpowering fear to leak away. He needed a small amount of time. He needed a little hope.

After that patient left for the hospital, Fred himself took me aside. He had overheard my parting comments in the hall and had surmised what had occurred. In his role as an "old hand" at AIDS in those horrific years, he was troubled by what I had told the once beautiful man that had just left my exam room. I had been wrong, Fred told me. Not just in this singular case, but in cases which might be like it. I should have told him everything, Fred believed, I should have told him that he had PCP, that he had AIDS, that he was dying. I listened to Fred and in my usual way didn't disagree immediately. But how and when to give the news was a vital part of medicine and I weighed his remarks carefully against my own perceptions and philosophy.

Those had been critical minutes in that exam room. In my careful words had laid the vortex of that man's existence—all of it spinning like ashes of his life swirling and falling like black snow. Was immediate complete truth always right? Was it better to give all information at once, even if the results of formal tests weren't completely known? I believe in being truthful with patients, but didn't the truth need to have a scientific basis, didn't we need to be certain? Or was experience and intuition sufficient for gut-wrenching pronouncement?

It was my normal practice to debate such disclosure; I had believed it was a judgment call whether to immediately speak the words of galloping inevitability or provide a merciful pause. Although this patient's chest X-ray was consistent with PCP, an unequivocal diagnosis couldn't be made from that alone. The man's HIV test and T-cell count, the definitive criteria, weren't yet known. It was our duty to be honest, but timing, I believe, depended on our assessment of the evidence and the individual. With this data ambiguous, should he have been told the journey to his death had begun, was I wrong that day? Had I postponed the news because I found it too difficult to deliver? Had I allowed my own feelings to come first? No, I reasoned, the data had not yet been established; my assessment was without laboratory findings. But with laboratory certainty, my experience had been that informing patients of the truth as soon as possible was best.

THE WORLD CRASHING DOWN

It's difficult to convey the sense of the world crashing down around us in those years of the late 1980s and early 1990s. Our staff was as susceptible to infection as our patients and we worked in an unsteady atmosphere of constant loss. Lawrence Medical rarely terminated office and medical assistants, but it wasn't uncommon for employees to leave the practice due to the emotionally overwhelming nature of our work. Unexpected losses were particularly disturbing—we were, after all, under siege and each disappearance was keenly felt. In spite of this environment, it was with surprise and consternation we learned one day that one of our assistants had been found dead in his car along the 405 freeway—a suicide unforeseen by our staff. I had barely known him.

Vincent was a gregarious man and so it was common to be meeting his new acquaintances. Two sports medicine physicians that he introduced to me were Tom and Stephen who were robust body builders. They had been partners outside the office but in spite of their separation their deprecating humor revealed their continuing affection for each other. They were especially engaging and, upon meeting them, Tom invited me and my Significant Other to his birthday party the following Saturday. Jack and I attended the event held at Tom's house in the Olympus sub-division of the city which, besides stunning views of the valleys below, had a large deck perfect for the party. The get-together was an elaborate affair with over 30 guests and both doctors dramatically wearing only white. The hors d'oeuvres were delicious and the toasts heartfelt.

But I had rare occasion to refer a patient for a sports medicine consult and I didn't interact with the two. It was a full six months later when I asked Vincent if he was seeing much of them. In spite of our work I was still surprised by Vincent's response: Stephen had succumbed three months after I met him and Tom had died the previous week. Vincent would be attending his funeral.

These were also times of grotesque irony. Phil and John weren't lovers, only room-mates, and were both seen by me. John, the older of the two, was a hypochondriac who did, at last, come into the office with a quarter-sized KS lesion on his neck. They had lived in hope they would never hear the bad news, but nevertheless feared it was in their future and the unfortunate day indeed arrived. Before John's KS lesion, his hypochondria had made him the focus of their joint attention which only skyrocketed after his diagnosis. His mother flew in from Philadelphia and we had multiple family conferences involving his mother, a brother in town and, of course, Phil. For a time I was receiving daily calls from either John or Phil concerning John's illness.

Six weeks after John's diagnosis, Phil called with fevers and a bad cough. I told him to meet me in the ER and there I discovered that his chest X-ray was "whited out." Although we started therapy immediately, and while he responded, he nevertheless died within a month. John, on the other hand, survived for another entire year.

In the last few months of 1990 the world truly seemed to be falling apart when I was asked to care for one of our own docs from the office. While staff deaths were deeply disconcerting, we had never had one of our physicians sicken. Luke Olson, M.D., had always looked gaunt in the way HIV makes one; he had the hallmark emaciation with prominent facial wasting and fat loss in the bi-temporal areas. Additionally, I had heard that Luke was "extraordinarily strange" from a staff member with whom he shared an apartment; however, I was to discover soon enough that it was something more than mere eccentricity.

Before I saw him Luke's condition had put him in the hospital where I was to interview and examine him. The door to his room had the usual patient's name with his Attending physician's name beneath it. As I brushed past the door, did I see "Olson/Dr. Faulk" or did I see "Faulk/Dr. Olson"? As I walked in the room, Luke was sitting up in bed with his hospital gown sagging with one side half undone. He was embarrassed—embarrassed to be hospitalized,

ANDREW M. FAULK, M.D.

embarrassed to be in a hospital gown, embarrassed to be in front of me. Embarrassed to be sick.

As I walked into the room, Luke sat with sunken temples and concave cheeks, sweating in a cold room, sipping water from a white styrofoam cup. I saw myself in that bed: gaunt, forlorn, needlessly ashamed. Here I was, examining a physician who had been my colleague only days before. As I sat down next to his bed, a new patient was rolled in to share his room which annoyed and distracted me. Many times Luke and I had sat across from each other in the LMG doctors' lounge, each working silently on our separate patient's charting. Here, with the chatter of nurses and patients banging around us, in the midst of one of the most sensitive conversations of our lives, we had neither quiet nor privacy.

He had been a professional confidant. Was I taking his medical history or was he taking mine?

Both of us felt awkward but it wasn't long before the details of his self-treatment spilled out of him like a penitent confessing to his priest. His diet had been strikingly different from that he had been recommending to his patients only days before. He had been a vegetarian, for how many months he couldn't remember. Almost always, in my experience, vegetarian diets in those with HIV lead to precipitous death due to the difficulty in getting enough nutrition and iron. Iron is complexed in red meat in such a way as to facilitate absorption in a manner that vegetables alone can't, especially, it seemed, in HIV malnutrition. But Luke's reason for excluding meat from his diet was one I had not heard before; he didn't eat meat because it made his urine especially disagreeable. In some East Indian tradition, Luke had been drinking his own urine. Refrigeration, he explained, made his urine more palatable. I could not imagine the consternation which our office assistant must have experienced when he first stumbled upon a supply of urine in his refrigerator.

My face remained expressionless. With people healthy one day and dead the next, disconnected families worrying about appearances, patients dying before their families even knew they were gay, people falling off radar only to be found dead next to busy freeways—all in a narcissistic society distant and apathetic. I was still surprised by Luke's admission. But whatever choices he'd made, I sat there without condemnation. Who was I to judge what paths someone took in attempt to escape the hangman's noose? In order to avoid some freak infection, Norman Nash hadn't simply rinsed his produce, his apples, oranges and peaches. He had diligently scrubbed them with soap and water. Luke had tried an unconventional, even bizarre, route to escape the juggernaut fast on his heels. Would some future doctor, safe in his or her world, sit in judgment of whatever decisions he had made? Perhaps the best personal maneuver, in the face of research that hadn't yet found treatment or cure, *was* to try various remedies, no matter how extraordinary or unlikely. Instead of waiting for the Scientific Method to wend its way to conclusion: a conclusion which could be answers or... silence. Instead of waiting for charts—statistics—studies—algorithms—numbers—diagrams, he had chosen to act. His particular choice had proven dreadfully misguided: in HIV depending on one's own urine for protein was tantamount to suicide. But what if his particular decision had been correct? I was waiting for scientific answers; he had not.

I watched as Luke, my co-worker, quickly succumbed in the following days. Between his inadequate diet and the ingestion of urine, he was extraordinarily malnourished, which hastened his death. I didn't have the time, or psychological energy, to mourn his death as I would have in a world less pressed with loss. The full expression of grief was a luxury I thought none of us had; emotional withdrawal was the only option. But Luke's passing pricked my professional detachment and drew blood.

BUSINESS AS USUAL
AS WE RUN INTO THE FIRE

It's difficult to describe the events of that period, to convey the crushing deluge of this terrible time. By the end of the 1980s, 90,000 people had died in the United States, hollowing out the gay communities of every major city before our eyes. To the world the crisis may have been invisible, but to us it was a war zone we lived in from which there was no respite. For me to endure, I thought, the horrible weight had to be managed, compartmentalized; I needed to shut down my emotions. But it was the nature of my psyche and the times that these walls of protection proved permeable at unexpected times.

One staff assistant, Carlos, had been a practicing physician in a Central American country, but was not licensed in the U.S. He was a quiet man but not because of any language barrier since his English was excellent. It was his job to usher patients in and out of exam rooms, so I was a little confused one day to find him remaining in a room with a patient, Michael—a man who had obviously been exceptionally handsome before HIV's assault. Even with the physical and psychological exhaustion that accompanies caring for someone with a terminal illness, Michael had become Carlos' lover.

But Michael's decline couldn't be stopped and we watched sadly as they fearlessly faced the end and moved in together. They only had a couple of months before he died, but in this instance atypical cracks in our emotional barricades allowed us to grieve with Carlos.

I didn't discuss my emotional detachment with anyone but it's clear now, looking back years later, that I calculated that the full expression of grief was a luxury that I didn't have and I shut down emotionally to protect that core in me that could still feel something.

It's clear to me now that a trained psychologist would've been of great help, but I seemed oblivious to the possibility of such a contribution. As our countrymen conducted business as usual, our office could lose as many as five or six patients a month, sometimes more, yet the world outside our walls seemed unaffected and untroubled. I was busy and yet I wasn't able to keep people from the edge, they were slipping off the earth and I was just giving them companionship along the way. I'd drive home, exhausted after a day of seeing patients, signing death certificates and taking calls from frantic patients or their families terrified about a lesion or desperate for information about any new treatment developments. Sometimes when I'd be washing my hands in some hospital room, I'd absent-mindedly ponder how someone my age should be out enjoying life, instead of inside writing orders for men I knew wouldn't live. We were the ones running into the fire, into the burning house, while others were running away from the flames—escaping to Palm Springs, to Bucks County, to Guerneville, or into mind-numbing jobs or unfulfilling relationships. Escaping the deluge of loss and grief and the burden of caring for those for whom it was too late to flee and from whom there was the horrific possibility of contracting the disease.

In society's neglect and opprobrium the government's budget for HIV research rose and fell, always staying absurdly small compared to the number of people dying. And too often families participated in this cover-up by hiding the deaths of their loved ones behind the words "pneumonia" and "cancer." On more than one occasion a brother or sister would plead with me not to disclose to a parent the reason for death, but ACT UP's war cry was bitter truth: "Silence Equals Death" and the accuracy of HIV statistics was too important to muddy. I told legal next-of-kin what I documented on death certificates; what was told to friends and relatives outside of these interactions was obviously outside of my control.

To me it is a mere technicality that President Ronald Reagan ("The Great Communicator") finally mentioned the word "AIDS" in 1985, for in the following years his lack of policy leadership was deadly: it rationalized minuscule research funding and fueled mainstream fear and hatred of gay men. His indifference reinforced the hostile zealotry of Evangelical Christians such as Jerry Falwell, who preached that "AIDS was the wrath of God on homosexuals."

Indeed Reagan's Communications Director, Pat Buchanan, stated that AIDS was "nature's revenge on gay men."

Thus the epidemic was confounded by a society which left us and our dying brothers largely abandoned and, initially, without services from kitchens to mortuaries. To their great credit it was the lesbian community as well as that of many heterosexual groups such as pockets of Catholic charities that jumped in—after their rejection of papal rules and sensibilities—to orchestrate AIDS fundraising, education and, that mark of true dedication and self-sacrifice, one-on-one care. They were the ones who, led by their sense of active compassion, began and staffed hospices, ran food delivery services to the house-bound and held the hand of the dying when their families shunned them. AIDS was catastrophic for the gay community and its supporters but, on the other hand, it frequently minimized our differences and bettered the world of the poor and sick.

MORNING DEATH LIST

After I had been at LMG for some time, we started making a list of those who had passed during the previous 24 hours. To learn of someone's death by chance in an overheard conversation in the hall or a receptionist's remark on the telephone was painful in its surprise—the sudden news unnerving, startling us and distracting us from our work. These deaths, while many were expected, wrought havoc with our emotions and created disruptions in the work until it occurred to me to prepare a list first thing in the morning. With this change in office procedure, each of us could read the list before work, and, in our own way, mark the passing of those patients we had cared for. Even if I didn't recognize the name, it was likely I had seen the person in clinic or hospital. On occasion, when a week seemed particularly heavy in losses, I would come into the office a half hour or so early. There would be bustling activity in the front reception area, but not in the back doctors' lounge (a 15' by 15' corner office with a large table in the center nearly filling the room). Sometimes another doctor had arrived before, but usually I would come in sufficiently early to find the lounge deserted and quiet. I would search out that single page before the sounds of the office grew to a distraction—perhaps I would ask one of the receptionists to print it if it wasn't already. Once I had the list, in the conference room I would brace myself by taking a quick glance at the number of names; afterwards I would read each entry more carefully. Perhaps it was someone I had seen last week, perhaps I had seen them only in the waiting room, but I knew them. The names better known would feel like a punch to my face, as if some heavy object struck my head. It was a rare day, however, that I would tear up—there were patients to be seen, other physicians to

ANDREW M. FAULK, M.D.

consult and lab numbers to evaluate. But when the week's losses were particularly numerous, or my connection to particular patients more intimate, I would leave the lounge and retreat into an empty exam room where I wouldn't be seen or disturbed, and silently stare at the white page heavy with names and, now, memories.

ACT UP

My feelings about the anarchic AIDS Coalition to Unleash Power (ACT UP) were always conflicted. On the one hand they were a welcome force in coalescing gay men, recruiting devoted lesbians, and heightening the awareness of the general public in their drive to force the government and drug companies to prioritize research and treatment, as well as pressuring the FDA to release drugs expeditiously. Their haunting triangle logo "Silence=Death" was genius in its truth, as was their use of the point-down pink triangle (used by the Nazis to identify gay people and, when superimposed on a yellow Star of David, simultaneously designated one as both homosexual and Jewish). While our brothers were dying all around us, ACT UP asked how those unaffected could continue on without any interruption in their lives.

At the same time indiscriminate targeting of the general public, including AIDS physicians and researchers, was mistaken. Apparently gay leaders from our recent history had been among the first fatalities and older, more seasoned, activists were largely replaced by those less experienced. I have always been a believer in the adage that one catches more flies with sugar than vinegar, and their techniques seemed heavily weighted on the side of vinegar. In June of 1990 I attended the International AIDS Conference held in San Francisco. Upon returning to the Moscone Center after lunch one day, my colleagues and I, clearly participants in the conference, were pelted by water balloons thrown by ACT UP members. We were some of those most dedicated to funding AIDS research and treatment, as well as expediting drug release and affordability. Obviously, to bombard us with water balloons was painfully misguided. Similarly

ANDREW M. FAULK, M.D.

I can see that blocking traffic on the Golden Gate Bridge during rush hour may have appeared to be the right thing to do in making our fellow citizens aware of our mounting losses. But San Franciscans were at the forefront of AIDS efforts and worsening traffic snarls for them gained us neither favor nor progress.

IN THE MIDST OF A WAR

At Lawrence Medical, for some time I served on call every third week and weekend. The on-call designate covered hospitalized patients with their great demand for consultation with specialists, families or significant others. It was a testament to Fred Lawrence's dedication and hands-on mindset that he himself was performing one-third of on-call coverage when I began. With the epidemic, Lawrence Medical had experienced an explosion of cases; physician workloads had skyrocketed long before I joined their practice. Vincent and Fred had worked tirelessly during the initial burst of AIDS as the practice grew exponentially. The growth of hours and our availability certainly was good for the budget but there also was a deep sense, shared by the entire office, that we were doing something of profound importance. We were functioning in a plague, in the midst of a war. Most doctors of the time either wouldn't treat HIV or didn't know how. On the other end of the spectrum were the purveyors of nonsense.

The years I was in practice had built a body of knowledge and experience that forswore the chasing of one medication or therapy after another. Especially in the early years of the epidemic, urgency and ignorance produced a wild rush for anything that offered a gleam of hope, and what I saw was sometimes amelioration and sometimes detriment. This provoked a profound skepticism in me about using untried medications. Although there was always the chance we were missing out on some new effective treatment, unless it was part of a study I came to believe there was no need to become crazy by chasing rumors.

We would hear of doctors who were practicing suboptimal medicine. And there were reports, backed by evidence, of some few

ANDREW M. FAULK, M.D.

M.D.s practicing a type of medicine which at best was incredibly poor judgment and at worst was an especially vicious form of fraud. The worst practitioners would treat their patients with Chinese herbs, acupuncture, Dale Carnegie positive thinking, Louise Hay visualization and camaraderie (e.g., "Hay rides") and various diets which were either vegetarian or some other nutrient-challenged diet. And then there were the "practitioners" who opted for various therapies based on "imbalances," methods of consumption, diet, mold or meditation alone. These charlatans and self-deceivers would "treat" these patients, my guys, until their condition was grave and then produce glowing statistics of homeopathic success by transferring them to us at the last minute for legitimate care by legitimate physicians.

Perhaps I spend too much time on my polemic against these people, but their destructive ignorance and magical thinking surrounded us and gave us at LMG another mission, a special mission. After presenting patients of these practitioners with the news of being HIV-positive or having an opportunistic infection, I would spend considerable time explaining that their lack of a positive attitude or visualizations were not to blame. You have a bad disease, I would repeat over and over. You are not responsible for all of this. With these kinds of pressures, it's easy to see we had a special calling. I am infected with HIV and my lifespan shortened, but my invaluable training was in the HIV wards of San Francisco themselves. Physicians have a special duty in times of crisis: I ran into the burning house, not away from it.

THE LOUISE HAY DAYS

Louise Hay was everywhere at the time. I never heard her speak, I never read a book she wrote, yet I dealt with her every day in my office. It may have been the EST movement which first started promoting the concept that people are responsible for all that happens to them. But what I constantly saw in my office was the belief system of Louise Hay which taught that those who are ill are ultimately responsible for their illness. When I saw Tom, or Ed, or Bill in the exam room, almost to a man they felt both sick and guilty. While I'm not by any means an authority in her various beliefs and practices, I saw the aftermath of her work, for what she taught landed front and center in those exam rooms on Wilshire Boulevard. One might imagine that, if there were fault, it was from whatever indiscretion had left my patients with the infection in the first place. No, that wasn't the guilt I dealt with every day in my office. My patients were struggling with the suffocating responsibility expressed in the ideas of Hay and her disciples.

Hay was born in 1926 and divined from a diagnosis of cervical cancer in 1977 or '78 that positive thinking could heal the body. She believed that forgiveness, therapy, nutrition, reflexology, and enemas were the route to healing; she authored several self-help books, the most influential being the 1984 book entitled *You Can Heal Your Life* ("If you can change your thinking you can change your life"). According to Louise Hay, in promoting this vision, she was the voice of a prophet in a sick and suffering world. That same year she began leading support groups in L.A. for people living with HIV which she called "Hay Rides." Those events grew from a few men in her living room to a large hall in West Hollywood. In March 1988,

ANDREW M. FAULK, M.D.

she was invited to appear on both "The Oprah Winfrey Show" and "Donahue."

How one views the various circumstances of life and how one constructs his life fundamentally affects his happiness, and happiness, I firmly believe, increases lifespan. Placebo and prayer, interestingly enough, have been shown to have an effect in fighting many cancers and conditions. In gauging the efficacy of prayer, it doesn't seem to matter whether the one who's praying is the patient or not, or whether the one praying has any degree of faith or religious commitment. Obviously one's attitude influences how one perceives his health. In every scientific experiment researching the efficacy of any medication or therapy, there's always a placebo; if the mind had no input into one's health, a placebo would be unnecessary.

Hay's New Age positive thinking may have given us insights into the benefits of affirmative thought, but the flip-side of this principle is a brutal insistence on personal accountability: if one can heal oneself, one can make oneself ill. If one says your thoughts can impact health, I agree. If one says your thoughts define your health, I disagree. I would deal with guilt—day after day, patient after patient—of those sitting in front of me who thought they were sick because they hadn't visualized good health with sufficient conviction or precision. They were ill because their imagery was incorrect or incomplete. A distraught patient, coughing, with a temperature of 103 degrees, and 110 pounds on a 6'1" frame, would "confess" that if only he had visualized properly he would not be in my office. If only he had believed enough. And some would draw the harsh conclusion from the extrapolation of Hay system logic that one is sick because they choose to be.

As I sat there, listening to the confessions of my misguided patients, I would curse the fatuous, sanctimonious teachings of the omnipresent Louise Hay. While dealing with the medical gravity of, say, *Pneumocystis jirovecii* pneumonia or Kaposi's Sarcoma, again and again I would need to begin by convincing my patients that imagination and visualizations, incantations and amulets couldn't provide protection against the virus. I battled daily with this crisis of my time and clan. In assisting my guys deal with death, I worked scrupulously to avoid religious or philosophical convictions, but here the wounds from their guilt were too damaging, the concepts too misguided. "You've got a bad disease," I would say, "you can't visualize it away; neither thinking nor belief can cure you." And then I would jump into what we knew of scientific treatment for their disease and symptoms.

ANDREW M. FAULK, M.D.

ADVICE, SELF-CARE, AND THE UNKNOWN

Besides being overwhelmed by their symptoms and guilt over supposedly shoddy visualization, my patients frequently felt that they needed to become medically educated overnight in order to survive their disease. Studies have shown a higher survival rate and greater happiness when patients are intimately involved in their own care. Before the Iron Curtain fell, global suicide rates were highest in Eastern Europe and it is commonly thought that they were a result of the lack of individual liberty. While it is optimal to be involved in one's own medical care, this can sometimes be confusing and overwhelming in a routine disease, let alone in the intricacies of a poorly-understood new retrovirus. Yet I was frequently awed by the command of the illness some "civilians" articulated. But this was a two-edged sword; a little knowledge is a dangerous thing. I've been at international AIDS conferences at which lay people have made extraordinarily perceptive suggestions and insights, and I have also heard remarks which showed little command of the scientific process and would've been incredibly destructive if acted upon.

"It's not your fault that you're becoming sick," I would say to my patients. "Even the most spiritually evolved person would get sick with what you have." My beginning statement was routinely needed because so many patients were caught up in the Louise Hay self-criticism meme. And then, judging by the response of the individual—especially listening to their choice of words—I would respond to their concerns.

The majority of people I saw took on the tremendous burden of getting the information necessary to play a proactive role in their own care. These were blue-collar workers and professionals of every stripe all suddenly overcome by this staggering avalanche of information. Most knew that proactive people did better, but they were confronted by a body of knowledge completely outside their experience. "I appreciate your wish to understand your problem," I would say. "And that's great. But you're attempting to educate yourself overnight about a newly-discovered, complex and poorly understood virus. It took me 11 years to become a doctor. You can't do the same thing in two weeks. You're asking too much of yourself. Find a doctor you trust—somebody you can be completely honest with. It might not be me and that's all right, but find the right doctor and relax in his or her care and stay up on HIV as much as you want. Or can."

Usually patients in this terribly painful initial period at first spoke of survival time. As always I would answer them that during any plague in human history a certain percentage of people would, as I would phrase it, "do well." It might be genetics, or self-care, or any number of factors, but there were always people that would "do okay" over the long-term. There was a chance, I would emphasize, that this person standing in front of me would do well.

If they spoke of needing to tell their loved one or their family of their sexual orientation, I offered my help—far too many families learned at the bedside.

Even though this was the message I gave my patients, I never included myself in the 10% survival rate I appeared to be seeing—a rate merely anecdotal and definitely not scientific. My motto, as was that of every doctor at LMG, was "Hope for the best. Plan for the worst." I didn't see myself living past 1993; it is the irony of my life that I have lived as long as I have. In 1993, I was certain I would step off the earth before 1995. And then in 1995 protease inhibitors came on the scene and changed everyone's arithmetic.

PROBLEM PATIENTS

Throughout my years of medical practice, I had a routine which was perhaps a bold-faced abuse of my position. Every year at Christmas I would discharge one patient from my practice. Of course this was done by legal procedure with registered notice and gave the individual ample time to locate another provider. It involved a number of registered letters with the recipient's signature required. A list of other acceptable doctors was always a nice touch, but not a requirement.

From my rogue's gallery of overly-demanding patients, there were those who were impossible to please, those who could only be satisfied with major sacrifices on my part. There is a relief, a tremendous relaxation, found in the recognition that you are human and cannot please everyone. Fred was not pleased with this custom I had carried with me from the dysfunctional San Francisco practice, but he nevertheless allowed this tampering with the practice—he recognized the pressure of our work.

So who was I to discharge from my practice and psyche? I had a small collection from which to choose. They fell into two clusters: the first, and by far the largest, were those whose passive-aggressive natures sabotaged my medical treatment and who loudly complained of my ineffectual management of their illnesses. The other, smaller group consisted of those incapable of recognizing my time and limitations. These were the "worried well," a group pointed out to us in medical school. Their sin lay in their trivial and petulant complaints which I could not help but compare to the desperate condition of their HIV-infected brothers. (I once received a call at 4 a.m. from one of these patients requesting a sleeping pill.) Those few patients we treated who were HIV-free knew full well the disease of the bulk of our patients. Had they been ignorant, their complaints and demands would have been easier to excuse. But they ignored the severity of disease around them which was, for me, exasperating. Had our modest fame not been known, a visit to our waiting room, with patients in various stages of serious illness, would have made our practice apparent. In addition, Fred and Vincent weren't shy about the field of our expertise. Advertisements, often full page and sometimes with photos, were strategically placed in the local gay newspaper. Tensions in a practice should be the last thing to influence doctor-patient interaction, but there it was.

UNDERSTANDING FRED LAWRENCE, M.D.

Before the epidemic, many gay doctors had slipped into only treating Sexually Transmitted Diseases (STD). It was, compared to other fields, remarkably uncomplicated. But once STD medicine morphed into HIV medicine and the epidemic began to monopolize our attention, many of these doctors retired. To his credit, Dr. Lawrence was one of those who had spent the time and energy to develop his expertise in treating the immunocompromised. He had learned it—as I had—from its beginnings, which was no small feat; as one doc told me with only a little hyperbole, "If you know HIV medicine, you know medicine."

Those patients who were also his long-standing friends certainly benefitted from his command of HIV medicine. But as time progressed, he gradually began transferring many of those patients to the care of Vincent and me. Fred was fond of repeating his personal maxim: "You don't need to be the best doctor, you just need to hire them." It was a compliment which made me smile inwardly every time I heard it, and perhaps revealed some of his thinking about those patients he transferred.

One of Fred's personal friends transferred to Vincent's care was Jeff Lysaght. Jeff was an extraordinarily engaging man with a somewhat eccentric handlebar mustache and ready remarks which displayed not only an intellectual prowess but also a command of the gallows humor in which we all participated from time to time. While he fell into my care only once or twice, it was more than enough to recognize him and hear his pungent remarks when we met in the LMG hallway as he headed toward Vincent's exam room. Jeff, in addition to whatever day job he held, volunteered at the annual gay rodeo held in nearby Burbank and it was always a pleasure to run into him, with his oversized mustache and his oversized wit, selling lottery tickets.

Although we were all too familiar with receiving random news at random times, I could not become used to hearing of the mounting deaths. While Jack and I had missed Jeff at the previous rodeo, as I had missed passing him in our halls, there had always been chance meetings and, besides, I didn't inquire of those I no longer saw. So it was with more than a little consternation that I heard of Jeff's death from Fred in that casual, unaffected manner. It seemed Jeff had succumbed to a pneumonia—perhaps PCP or some other bacteria or virus in which the immunocompetent among us swim with unconscious impunity.

"Jeff was always afraid of drowning," Fred told me, "I guess in the end that's how he died." Fred and I were in his Mercedes driving home from one of our monthly office meetings. These get-togethers were held in a variety of restaurants with the tab, of course, being picked up by the office. As a remnant of the frugality of my life during the years of training, this felt like a grand luxury. During that particular business meeting, I had ordered a cocktail. I had thought little of it, although the gathering was devoted to the running of the office. In Fred's car, however, before he gave me the news about Jeff, he reprimanded me for the drink. In the darkness, I felt myself blushing. It was one innocent drink, but in my ridiculously hyperactive conscience the failing was as large as a missed laboratory test result.

As I pushed that discomfort out of my mind, he told me the news about Jeff's pneumonia and death. As usual, however, when discussing the passing of any of his friends or patients, his tone of voice was one of detached, resigned acceptance. But after the news, I was shocked when his hand reached across the car's console to the passenger's side where I was sitting and grasped my hand. His left hand remained on the steering wheel as he held my hand with his right. He continued driving in his usual terrifyingly high speed which had earned him multiple tickets and traffic school classes (although I strongly suspected that he arranged for others to attend these mandatory driving schools). With a little reflection, I considered that while I may have chosen a cocktail, Fred chose to drive like a bat out of hell.

That night he held my hand in the car for what seemed like an eternity. Maybe it was an eternity. In spite of the emotional care I routinely gave my patients, I was uncomfortable. I was ashamed of my discomfort, but then again, I was sitting in my boss' car as he held my hand. Realizing that the extreme, the terrible, nature of our work had evidently hit his heart, I relaxed. The world was upside-down—nothing was normal, nothing was abnormal.

PHYSICIAN-ASSISTED SUICIDE
AND GOODBYE PARTIES

During my first years in San Francisco in the 1980s, I attended a going-away party for a tall, thin man who was obviously ill. He was a member of a gay social club in the city and, instead of remaining in San Francisco, had decided to spend his last days back where he grew up in central Pennsylvania. I was unaccustomed to such a send-off with its crushing heaviness. But as the epidemic ground on, farewells became more immediate and heart-wrenching as the community became familiar with both the devastating course of the disease and the possibility of actively controlling the timing of one's own death.

During my time of practice in L.A., I attended the "Goodbye Parties" of three of my patients and one of an acquaintance which were all far more intimate and heart-breaking than the send-off I had attended during those earliest years of the epidemic. All three of my patients had had partners and many friends who had preceded them in death and who had shown them, by example, the unkind end which the disease could bring. I had long talks with each. Most patients who consider physician-assisted suicide do so out of fear of uncontrolled pain and destruction of autonomy and, while I could assure them they could expect scrupulous pain management from me, I couldn't address issues of loss of independence outside of a metaphysical discussion. When we deal with the loss of physical independence, can't we perhaps consider this a potential lesson in humility for ourselves and possible emotional growth for our loved ones and care-givers? Despite the strength or weakness in these arguments, all three feared obliteration of control over their own bodies and remained firm in the decision to end their lives. I found

ANDREW M. FAULK, M.D.

it overwhelmingly difficult to argue that such a fundamental choice shouldn't be their own. In keeping with accepted standards in those states and countries where physician-assisted suicide is legal, I sent each to a doctor outside of LMG to confirm that they had no more than six months to live, and also to an associate psychiatrist to rule out depression or dementia.

These three chose the time of their death before the disease chose it for them. They had decided to make the end of their life a celebration; two of the three maxed out their credit cards renting expensive hotel suites, having a DJ, providing an open bar, and catering food. One was in the Hotel Sofitel in L.A., a venue not as plush as its cost. As disturbing as it was to attend any of these "parties," I felt it was my responsibility—it was my signature, after all, on the prescription. F. Scott Fitzgerald wrote in *The Great Gatsby*, "Let us learn to show our friendship for a man when he is alive and not after he is dead." Attending Goodbye Parties, as incredibly heartbreaking as they were, was truly showing friendship for a man "when he is alive."

The capacity of anyone to come to grips with one's own impending death, I have found, has little to do with his capabilities in other parts of his life. We all are mortal, so why is it such surprise to face our end? Certainly I know first hand this situation, I can be enjoying some trivial pleasure when the razor blade of awareness draws blood. Just when I think I've come to grips with my own death, a small thought throws me back to where I started. It is a veritable onion of feelings: right when I think I've finished peeling off the skin, another layer appears. As I turn my head toward some little pleasure of life, my mortality can slap me in the face.

As with most all of my practice, I didn't discuss Goodbye Parties with Jack. I kept these emotions to myself and dealt with them alone.

Thomas "Jerry" Bingham usually came into my office with one of two friends, either Kurt or Jim. The lines on his face, together with his longish greying hair, identified him in my mind as an aging hippie. He often teased me about the formality of my white lab coat over a shirt and tie. During many of my years in medicine I tended to look younger than I was and so, in my struggle to gain credibility, traditional medical clothing seemed best. But once I realized that connectedness was at the heart of what I could give my patients, I removed my coat and tie and unbuttoned my shirt.

Unhappily Jerry had between 100 and 200 T-cells and his visits with me had us watching their relentless drift downward as the disease progressed. His manner was bright, however, and he had that rare motivation, insight, and grace with which some patients make the physician feel better, rather than vice versa. As his T-cells dropped below 200, I placed him on pentamidine, an antibiotic commonly used to treat and protect against PCP, the AIDS-related pneumonia.

Lawrence Medical did not assume the care of those without private insurance of some kind. But if a patient lost their coverage while under our care, they were never discharged from our practice. "Once a patient, always a patient" was the motto of Lawrence Medical and it was a philosophy that met my own sensibilities and ethics. Truth be told, I'd have preferred a practice which took everyone regardless of their insurance status, but losing one's insurance was frequent and we ended up treating many patients *gratis*. No matter his insurance, Jerry's care with us was secure. Our finance department, however, let me know his non-Medicaid insurance had collapsed and, more importantly, he was running out of money for non-medical expenses, although they were working with him on acquiring funds from AIDS Project Los Angeles (APLA). At various visits Jerry and I discussed his situation with Kurt and Jim. Kurt had offered Jerry a place to stay, but Kurt's finances were equally dire. And Jim had space constraints of his own.

In spite of these impediments, Jerry didn't seem to be depressed—just running out of options that he found acceptable. Unfortunately, he was one of the many to have extensive facial KS lesions and with each office visit there were more. Jerry began to envision a future similar to that of those he knew who had passed before him, a future bereft of those things which made him happy. Kurt was with him in my office when he proposed a doctor-assisted suicide. Not in those words, of course.

"Hey, Doc, can you give me something to make it all go away?" I answered, "We're giving you everything we can, Jerry." He said, "No, Dr. Faulk, I mean everything." My eyes shot a glance to Kurt. "What do you mean exactly, Jerry?"

"I've lived a lot of good years, and all the ones ahead look bad. There are more KS lesions all the time and I can't look at myself in a mirror; I'm too embarrassed to leave my house. Can't you give me something to make me go to sleep?"

"Jerry, do you know what you're asking? Maybe another visit with our psychiatrist, Dr. Samuels, will help."

"I'm not depressed, Doc. I just don't want to go down the path that Mark did." (Mark had been his partner who had died two years earlier.)

"Well, I want you to really think about this. Do me a favor and see if APLA can't provide a different living situation. And why not see Samuels again?"

"I've thought about it already, Dr. Faulk, and I just don't want any more appointments. I like Dr. Samuels but the meds I'm on aren't changing my mind. I'm not sad. I'm just tired and I don't like what I see ahead of me."

We discussed this over a period of a month, but I asked him to make another appointment to see me in two weeks. After Jerry left my office, I called Martin Baines, our financial department's whiz kid. He told me that he had already spoken to Jerry about a number of possibilities and APLA had offered him their social workers and other county options which Jerry hadn't pursued. Peter Samuels, our psychologist, confirmed that Jerry wasn't depressed, just facing a grim future.

The next time I saw Jerry, both Kurt and Jim were with him. They confirmed that Jerry didn't seem depressed—just running out of alternatives.

His time ahead looked as bleak to me as it did to him, but my role was to give him as much encouragement as I could. I asked him to make one more appointment with our consulting psychiatrist—but I wrote him out the script just the same. The piece of paper seemed too small for what it could do. As I handed it to Jerry, I repeated my standard line for this situation, "Jerry, whatever you do, don't take all the pills at once and chase it with a fifth of gin."

In less than a week I heard back from our psychiatrist and Martin. Their evaluations had not changed. Jerry wasn't clinically depressed and APLA had discovered several housing options. That same day, however, Jerry called me on the phone. As they disrupted my schedule, I rarely took non-emergency calls during my workday; either I returned calls in the morning before I had seen my first patient or after I had seen my last. But I quickly took Jerry's call.

"Andrew," Jerry said, addressing me for the first time by my given name, "Kurt, Jim and I are having a little going away party on Sunday and it'd mean a lot to me if you could come."

"Are you sure you want to do this, Jerry?" I felt a chill run down my back.

"Yeah, I don't want to see what I see in the mirror anymore. I'm at rest with things going like this."

As I worked in our office on Saturdays, Sunday was a day I was available. Unlike most other goodbye parties, Jerry's send-off was not a lavish, extravagant affair—he evidently had never been in a position to nurture credit cards. So instead of the more costly hotel suite, Jerry had his send-off at home.

He lived in a small ranch house in the San Fernando Valley heavily shaded by trees and, unlike the majority of his neighbors, a yard off to the side. Jerry's bedroom opened directly onto this large side-yard and he had moved his mattress from a bed to the floor in front of the doorway. For the most part, he remained on the mattress, legs folded into a lotus position. His roommates had set up a folding table outside with jug-wine, a few bottles of different liquors, and plastic cups. Jerry stayed on the mattress with the door open to the others, as his few visitors, with plastic cups in their hands, drifted between the bedroom and the yard. It was a warm day in the valley but not as horrendously hot as was common and I was thankful for the trees. In the living room a cheap stereo played a collection of rock pieces from the late 1970s and early '80s. All the windows of the house were open, and the music could easily be heard throughout the yard and house. I recognized one other patient of mine in the little group that had formed and greeted him, awkwardly, and talked with him a bit. Although everyone attending knew the purpose of the get-together, Jerry had been diplomatically circumspect about where the prescription had come from. At one point, one of the strangers asked me if I had written it. I answered him that he would have to ask Jerry.

Someone had brought orange juice which one or two of the guests mixed with vodka and which I preferred to the jug-wine. There were five or six people there when I arrived and the number grew no bigger than ten.

About half of his guests, in sitting with Jerry, teared up but it was a period in my life in which I didn't cry (Jack had not yet died) and I was thankful that keeping a dry eye wasn't a struggle for me. There were few conversations in the yard among this somber group. But there at the doorstep, the conversations with Jerry, more often than not, were of common remembrances of various shared events. Once again I was struck by the comforting power of connection—connection which I now saw as crucial to patient care.

Jerry appeared determined and at peace with what was going to conclude the day. "Thanks, Dr. Faulk, for making this get-together possible." In spite of his intent, I found his comment disturbing. I could make this decision for myself, but what about my signature on Jerry's prescription? I had sworn the oath of physicians throughout history: *primum non nocere*—first, do no harm. My promise was to do what was best for those who had entrusted me with their well-being. Was I doing the right thing? Was this doing ultimate harm rather than ultimate good?

Repeatedly I spoke to him about the "cocktail" he was about to take.

"Jerry, you can change your mind at any time," I said. "If you do, tell Kurt or Jim and we'll have you hospitalized right away. Depending on the timing, it's likely that we'll have a good chance of success."

I imagined myself in Jerry's place. Should he change his mind at any point, I didn't want him to feel trapped by inertia or embarrassment. He was not to die in panic, no matter how far the medications had progressed. "I'm only a phone call away," I emphasized. I knew I'd be spending the rest of the afternoon and evening next to my phone. I calmed myself—should it come to that, I'd be able to more or less control emergency intervention as I knew which drugs were involved.

"No, Dr. Faulk, that won't happen. I won't be needing your services any more." Jerry's formality reinforced my heavy responsibility. "But I thank you for all the help you've been to me; you were always there when I needed you. You're a good man."

I probably spent 30 minutes sitting on Jerry's doorway stoop while he reclined a few feet away on the mattress. Out in the yard Kurt and Jim quietly thanked me but their gratitude provoked mixed emotions. My prescription would kill my patient; handwriting on a piece of paper would end Jerry's life. My handwriting.

Finally I left the gathering—that little, modest accumulation of his closest friends and few possessions. If I were him, would I have chosen this clean break, this simple walk to the edge? Could I swallow all those pills knowing that they would carry me off the earth? To know the possible course of a disease isn't the same as knowing with certainty how it would evolve in a specific person. Neither Jerry nor I knew how AIDS might progress in his case.

When someone was newly diagnosed with HIV, I'd tell them the scientific truth: that in any epidemic there were a percentage who survived. Any one patient might be on the positive side of the statistical bell curve. There was always a chance, I would tell my patients, there was always a possibility they would be one of those to survive.

At this point in my career, I'd only seen two long-term survivors, and one of them was me. Nevertheless, the hope I encouraged in my patients, I didn't entertain in myself. To give myself hope felt too much like fooling myself. Was I to be the exception, after all? Unlikely. If I had any number of malignancies, I calculated, my odds would have been better.

But had I projected my internal hopelessness onto Jerry? Would he have been one to actually survive the epidemic?

When my time comes, I hope I have the grace to accept death— but I make no promises. It may well be that I won't be able to accept my approaching fate. But I hope that I will confront death with the same courage demonstrated to me so often in those patients with whom I've walked to the edge of the world.

ANDREW M. FAULK, M.D.

MARK RAUCH'S LETTER

In the last week of the life of my patient Mark Rauch, he wrote this letter to my team and me. From his hospital bed, and in his great illness, concentrating and writing this must have been a terrific burden. But one morning on rounds that last week, he handed this to me. I knew my parents understood my practicing medicine, but I wasn't sure they realized the breadth of my work. I mailed them a copy of his letter followed by a note home:

The first time I was hospitalized I watched a lot of television. Most of it was dreadful. One show I enjoyed was "All in the Family." To be most precise, I enjoyed watching Edith. In hospitals there is much time to think and I thought about why I was so affected by this character called Edith. She wasn't pretty, or smart, or witty. She accomplished nothing that history would record. Her days were spent caring for her family.

Edith cared. Edith did more than care, Edith loved. That was what made her real for me. She had that which can create paradise out of hell; she had that without which all is awful—she loved uncritically all who came into her life.

Edith was only a character on a show, but I've known people like her. And it is to these people I wish to say "Thank you." You have comforted me in my despair, washed me, combed my hair, done my laundry. The world may never know of your kindness, but I know, and when I stand before God, your names will echo through the throne room in praise until all the angels take up the cry, then will the universe tremble, and in its secret places write your names, but nowhere will they be engraved more deeply than in my heart.

You had but little you could give, yet you gave it. Great achievements were beyond you, yet you waged endless war against despair and fear. The get well card, the phone call, the visit you made, changed my life. I do not exaggerate. I could be dying alone, hopeless and unloved. Because of you, I die surrounded by love and I die loving you—the unseen saints of this earth.

You have comforted me, now may I comfort you. Pain shall pass, grief shall be forgotten. Love endures, and one day, be assured, the circle will be unbroken. Lift up your hearts.

Mark E. Rauch
Summer 1954—Autumn 1988

Dear Mom & Dad,
Mark died under my care Nov. 16 and wrote this letter to his doctors before he passed away (The dates at the bottom are his own). This is what I do. This is what I do for a living. I love you both. —Andrew

ANDREW M. FAULK, M.D.

PHYSICIANS, NOT PRIESTS

Many of my patients knew their prognosis as soon as they got an AIDS diagnosis (the formal determination of AIDS requiring both a positive HIV test as well as an opportunistic infection or T-cells below 200), but a significant number of them had lived in isolation from others with the disease, as Dr. Mark Higgins has remarked, and were unacquainted with the illness. I learned that it was best to inform these men of their diagnosis and the usual course of the disease as soon as possible since their learning this from some overheard, casual comment would have been brutal. To keep the patient uninformed, or half informed, was tantamount to a lie that would have made it impossible to create a real connection. Besides, withholding or delaying information would have been an act of condescension since it assumed they were unable to constructively process the information.

When it came to supplying the necessary details about their prognoses, I saw my function as nearly that of a technician plainly giving unadulterated test results. (Precise life-span was almost always unknown and therefore rarely discussed.) In the beginning of my practice, I worried that I destroyed hope when I delivered the necessary information. But I found that, whatever hope was lost and no matter the initial devastation, men who had more facts faced their end better in the long run—they seemed to experience less crippling terror and depression than I might have expected. I saw that embracing clear truth gave them an opportunity to face the totality of their lives and reach past a point of old grudges and allow forgiveness. Informing my patients was better than not; knowing was better than not knowing.

And if a patient remarked on his personal beliefs, if he introduced the subject, I would encourage him to elaborate on his spiritual views. My listening to the details of their convictions went a long way in making my patients feel understood and respected; moreover, actively listening expanded my grasp of their social web, their sensibilities, and their priorities. Conversation built connection. In being heard, my patients became full participants in medical and social decisions.

In order to be free to discuss these issues without prejudice, however, I had to try to bury my own convictions and reject any temptation to introduce my own spiritual notions. If a patient feels that his doctor is uncomfortable discussing spiritual beliefs, dialogue will be damaged and support shortchanged. When I interrupted conversation, I may have made myself feel more comfortable, but not my patient.

I can't really explain why some patients seemed to experience a larger measure of quiet, of calm, sometimes even those in whom I would have expected more anguish and chaos. Other than working for connectedness, I certainly don't credit myself for any serenity my men may have achieved. I was merely a stepping stone in their journey. After all I was a physician, not a priest.

A PATIENT'S FUNERAL

During those years I attended only one funeral of a patient. I had known Harry Johnson better than most and I felt compelled to say goodbye. The world had lost someone valuable when it lost Harry and I wanted the opportunity to mark the sad passing with those who loved him. Harry and his partner, David, had many friends and his parents and sister had been wonderfully supportive—it was to be a large funeral. Once I arrived at the church, I was startled to find myself in a sea of black dresses and dark suits. I didn't own a suit and I cursed my lack of planning; I was an AIDS doctor after all, it was absurd for me not to own a black funeral suit.

I sat on the aisle in the back row. There were a number of other patients there, but my presence was noticed only by one or two. I was struck by a paranoid, fleeting thought that somehow I would be identified as responsible for Harry's death.

In the center of a busy hallway in the North Hollywood hospital, a patient's brother had once screamed that I'd killed his brother (by ordering a C.T. scan). This same brother had been homophobic toward the patient and routinely excluded him from family gatherings. And yet it was his ostracizing brother who had loudly called me a murderer that day. It was my sad experience that frequently those who were the most critical of a patient's care were actually the most distanced. It's often the uninvolved mother, the critical brother, the judgmental father, the hyper-religious sister who criticizes a patient's care the most. I don't want to undervalue this man's grief, but this kind of reaction—usually on a lesser scale—was not uncommon in some family members.

But I knew, of course, Harry's family had loved him profoundly and I had treated him until there had been nothing more to do. As those present, perhaps 200, all took their seats, I realized I was feeling uncomfortable and it had nothing to do with my clothing. I was troubled by the knowledge that I knew Harry far more intimately than most of those sitting in the pews. I had been with him through his presenting pneumonia and had identified the first lesion on his back as KS. I was there when Harry was tormented by thoughts of the grief he would cause David and I had been there when David pulled me out into a hospital hall and wept with his impotence and fatigue. I had known Harry very, very well in the last few months of his life—I was part of this group of mourners but strangely not. In spite of the deepest emotional connection, or because of it, I was outside this group of grieving people.

Somewhere in the service, the reverend asked for anyone who had something to say, a memory perhaps, to stand and speak. Without a significant pause, several people got up and shared a memory aloud and I was surprised to learn of several details of his life I hadn't known. Finally there was a pause as the reverend awaited other remarks. The seconds seemed like minutes as I wrestled with myself whether I should stand and speak. There was so much that could be said: from Harry's bravery to his love for David. But this was not about me, I reasoned—the attention was to be on Harry's life. I imagined my mother, however, who delighted in recounting drama and who would have reported how touching it was for the doctor himself to stand and speak. These feelings finally won out and just as I was about to stand, the interval ended. Part of me was relieved as I am not a public speaker, but another part was disappointed that my hesitation would mean Harry's gathered friends and relatives would not hear my few remarks, my few observations. And his mother wouldn't be able to say afterwards that even his doctor had stood to eulogize her son.

CANCER AT THE FRONT DOOR

In September of 1990, Jack developed a painless lesion in the back of his throat which he felt when he swallowed. I wish I had accompanied him to UCLA hospital the day he was examined, but the fact was that the problem didn't register with me, somehow, that it could have been something serious. It should have—we had known since his pneumonia in 1987 that he was immunocompromised and therefore my tranquility was rooted in denial. For me it was unthinkable that Jack might be up against one of those punishing diseases I saw in my office every day.

When he returned I was in my upstairs study—my "man-cave"—when I heard him slam the door. "I have cancer," I heard him yell. There was neither a remark before nor after. Just "I have cancer." I ran down the stairs. Yes, I had heard correctly. I could see the shock on his face as I had heard it in his voice. There was no manufactured distress that day, no faux horror to break the deathly seriousness of the moment as there had been at S.F. General those years before. This felt more serious than that, as it was. He didn't bawl then, his face didn't crinkle into a mask of play weeping as it did when he was clowning. Rather, his face remained motionless as tears silently wet his cheeks.

Jack "clucked," in his normal fashion meaning: "this is what it is and I'll have to get used to it."

"Hey," I said. "This isn't all there is, there are things we can do." I grabbed his neck, and pressed my forehead to his.

After nine months of chemotherapy, Jack passed away no more than 10 feet from where we stood that day.

"IT'S NOT SUPPOSED TO HAPPEN
TO A DOCTOR"

I was interviewed in the fall of 1990, anonymously, for an article that appeared in the October 7, 1991, *L.A.C.M.A. Physician* (Los Angeles County Medical Association periodical). Tom Jennings was the author of the article entitled "It's Not Supposed to Happen to a Doctor." In it, I said I expected to be out of my practice in two years, dead in four. I told him, "What I've come to realize is that this is a lethal disease and it is going to take my life." But I also expressed surprise that I was doing so well. The CDC study, in which I remain an active subject, sees me about three times a year. A few years later, one of the researchers who was examining me suggested that my strain of HIV could be particularly weak; this may or may not be so, but what I did have was a missing CCR5 gene—an absence found most often in those of Northern European descent. In most people, this gene produces proteins on the surface of lymphocytes which effectively work as one of several "doors" for HIV entry. Without that gene's proteins, my lymphocytes have one less point of entry for the virus. There are still many other points of entry for the virus, obviously, so I'm not immune.

Tom Jennings began his interview:

"Physicians seemed to have it all. He was young, he had a lucrative practice—and he had HIV. Now he talks, anonymously, about fear and prejudice in the medical community, and how that attitude must change."

Here are a few of the comments I made:

"I have seen many nurses and even physicians treating their HIV-positive patients in an inappropriate manner. I've seen nurses

ANDREW M. FAULK, M.D.

gown up and put on gloves to simply interview an AIDS patient. That is very distressing to the patient and is not based on scientific fact, but strictly on emotions. That does nothing for the patient's sense of well being and self respect...

"It makes me furious when I hear people like Senator Jesse Helms saying that spending for AIDS is out of proportion to other life-threatening illnesses. What he fails to take into account is the man-years that are lost when a young person dies rather than an elderly person. If a grandmother who has heart failure dies, although it's tragic in its own right, society is not losing the productivity a 35-year old has to offer...

"I believe that HIV will eventually be curable and even prevented with vaccines. When that will happen, I don't know. I'm pessimistic that I will live to see it happen. Like I tell my patients: hope for the best, plan for the worst."

OUR DENIAL

Although we talked about our visits to the chemotherapy clinic and my anti-nausea cocktail, in that last year I took my cues from Jack and didn't discuss his death. Nor did we talk about any doubts he may have had about the chemotherapy he took for the last nine months of his life. He never asked me the percentage of those treated who survived long-term. (In those times, almost all patients with HIV-related non-Hodgkins lymphoma succumbed well within the first year.) When he was first hospitalized with PCP in San Francisco, he listened quietly when his father pressed him to do physical exercises, but he knew that his was a far more serious disease than could be treated by simple bed exercises. Despite Jack's opting for every medical treatment available, his clucking revealed his growing pessimism.

I spent much of my professional energies helping others work through their denial. Once the energy supporting denial was refocused, my patients frequently had more honesty and forgiveness with their loved ones and often a less troubled end. Randy Shilts, the great chronicler of the epidemic, wrote that his life was finished without being complete—my goal was to assist as many as I could in finding their lives were complete. It was the paradox of my life that as my practice became increasingly specialized in helping patients accept reality and walking with them the last steps of their lives, I didn't find this kind of success at home. But the truth was that I didn't employ my abilities; I simply couldn't be Jack's physician. People frequently lose their professional strengths once they're no longer functioning in their usual capacity and this was what occurred with me. For I was not his physician—I was his husband—and I simply didn't fit or want another role. The reality was I had my own denial and he may well have received signals from me that denied his mortality; I had, after all, conjured a thousand ways for him to live to be 80. Engulfed by his own denial, I wanted to believe that in his preternatural innocence, in his tenacious happiness, he would survive. So in addition to my professional limitations, I wrestled with my own reluctance to accept the inevitable.

The day before he died he asked me what drug we would use next. As a doctor I said nothing, as a husband I told the lie that there was yet another option. But there was no remaining treatment.

MAKING A HOSPITAL ROOM HOME

Each time Jack was hospitalized I bought a poster for him and had it professionally framed—a serene poster, something full of colors that soothed the eye and heart. It would be a finished piece of art, attractive enough to hang in our home. But first it would keep him company in the hospital, something to look at that wasn't institutional. I would hang it in his room, nail and hanger, regardless of the nurses' reluctance or hospital regulations. It would hang on each facility's wall, under harsh lighting, among voices of command and acquiescence in the early morning hours, there in the late afternoon hours when the sunlight is harsh and unforgiving and then again before dusk fell. He would have something homey then and something of me to tell him he wasn't alone whether it be three in the morning or three in the afternoon. During those afternoon hours it is unseemly for death to occur, but the relentless clock nevertheless works its way into the very early morning hours—2 a.m. or 3 a.m.—in which it is more seemly, more expected somehow, for death to come. And when he came home there would be something new to hang in the house. It was not unlike the child mollified with candy after the doctor's poking and prodding… morphed into something more adult-sized, yet just as comforting. After its time on the wall, the artwork would stay with us and I'd make room for it at home. So Jack would be wheel-chaired out of the hospital, in unforgiving hospital gowns, with a carefully framed print balanced on his knees, a souvenir that became part of our shared consciousness.

ANDREW M. FAULK, M.D.

JACK'S CHEMOTHERAPY—
THE THURSDAY ROUTINE

Jack had chemotherapy every Thursday until the last few weeks of his life when all treatment was futile. In my overheated schedule as physician and primary caregiver, this was one of the two days in my week that belonged to me. At LMG, I changed my schedule to Monday through Wednesday and Friday and Saturday. In addition I served as on-call physician one week out of every four or five. On the weekends the on-call designate also covered hospital rounds, with its greater demand for consultation with specialists, and meetings with families and significant others. The on-call M.D., on occasion, might be asked to round on all the hospitalized LMG patients. During the last year of my practice, I found myself being asked to do more and more hospital work as opposed to office/clinic work. My insecurities made me a detail man, and thus good for those patients whose medical complexity was escalating or those whose illness was sufficiently serious to require hospitalization. We had a reputation for treating AIDS patients well—not just from a cutting edge, up-to-the-minute scientific perspective, but also from a psychological/emotional point of view. "You don't have to be the smartest doctor, you just have to hire the smartest doctor." I was keenly aware of how little we knew about the disease, and it was this insecurity that was significantly responsible for my professional drive. But Fred and Vincent had another reason for shunting me more and more to the hospital. My colleagues could depend on my ability to treat people medically—and emotionally—at the very worst moments of their lives. In our efforts to connect with people, our most powerful tool is empathy and my life story and my own HIV status, while undisclosed, gave me an empathy which translated into an ease in achieving that all-important connectedness. And while my history and HIV status wasn't known or stated explicitly, I believe my patients felt my willingness to face my own similar fears on common ground with them. They could appreciate this all-important connectedness; we were in this together. So I was spending more and more of my time rounding in the hospital and taking weekend calls.

I was incredibly grateful that there was not a word of complaint from anyone in the office when I began to take every Thursday off to be with Jack for his chemotherapy. We would get up together on those days and have a breakfast of something bland like yogurt and cereal. Jack would have his tea just the way he liked it and I would have my coffee. I'd carefully watch the clock so we wouldn't be rushing as we drove to UCLA hospital. There we would park in their below-ground parking and find our way to the outpatient treatment. After signing in and sitting down in an attractive waiting room, we would search the tables for anything which would distract us a bit from the other patients waiting for chemotherapy and our approaching treatment. During those first months the sight of our thin co-travelers with their haunted eyes and tell-tale turbans and baseball caps would hit us like a bucket of cold water. But after some five or six weeks of therapy, the shock of their appearance melted away and we began seeing them as the three-dimensional people they were.

Jack, who found silence to be deadly and individual relationships engrossing, would frequently strike up a conversation and find hope in the worst case scenarios. I, on the other hand, found it difficult to relax and challenging to engage other patients in conversation. No matter. Although occasionally nervous, Jack fulfilled his role as the consummate party thrower. The eternal mingler, he would tease out their stories while, unexpectedly, keeping silent about much of his own. A beautiful 23-year-old woman with brain cancer answered Jack's sympathetic questioning, "Oh, I was cancer-free for six months and I'm back again." She produced pictures of her cat playing, and reported that the cat was pregnant and she hoped to live long enough to see the birthing. The others in the waiting room were a different group of people: middle-aged women with breast cancer, less well-kept older men who appeared blue collar with prostate cancer, and the occasional young person in their early 20s or 30s with a heavy metal band on their T-shirt. This last group, the younger ones, would haunt my thoughts for days after we were back at home—had they already seen the best days of their lives?

It seemed that most patients came alone, but there were many who came accompanied. Some barely spoke but they all had their own life story and through the random remarks and more serious discussions we caught glimpses of their pressured lives. It was a time together that could make us feel good about ourselves, our doctors and our conditions one week, and then be desperately depressed the next. I would like to say that because of my daily work, I wasn't negatively affected by this group with different cancers and different attitudes, but their haggard, run-down appearance did everything but convince me that cures were right around the corner for any of us. And once it became clearer that Jack wasn't doing as well as we hoped, he slipped into the role of happy interviewer less and less.

When they called Jack's name, we'd walk into the chemotherapy suite and I would sit him down in one of the hyper-comfortable lounge chairs which UCLA had specifically for this purpose. Each chair was its own little alcove, its own niche, although there was little actual privacy owing to the constellation of some 20 other chairs on each side and across the large room; but it was a cheerful place with big picture windows looking out onto a green lawn. One could not ask for better nurses—they were patient, competent and reasonably cheerful. I would hold Jack's hand while they found a cooperative vein and sit there while the medication dripped into him. Always the comedian Jack would make comic observations of the nurses attending him, sometimes within their hearing, sometimes not. But the real targets of his remarks, albeit unknown to them, were the other patients in their own, separate, little cubicles. Those around us seldom knew his insightful remarks or his uncanny witticisms, but had his observations been overheard, I suspect most patients as well as bystanders would have laughed in recognition and agreement. Though they may not have known it, Jack was an ally.

I deeply appreciated UCLA's gesture at providing something of the natural world to look at. Those facing severe illnesses gain so much from an open window or an open door. It seems the valuable effects of nature are multiplied in those debilitated sick who face the sterile world of windows that don't open and rain that can't be heard. Getting outside into nature, even if it's just the grass of a backyard, can recharge and refocus our energies. Music, too, is of incomparable value—it can give us access to words and worlds that are lost in the all-consuming distillation of one's attention that a fatal illness produces. Music uncovers and articulates those emotions which need to be expressed and it may be one of the few pleasures that one is still able to remember and experience. Auditory memories from long ago can comfort us and music can remind us we are alive. Oliver Sacks writes of "a deep and mysterious paradox here, for while music makes one experience pain and grief more intensely, it brings solace and consolation at the same time." Many of my patients responded to music with a serenity they seemed to find nowhere else.

We must help people live their lives as fully and as long as they are able.

I will never know for sure if Jack was one of those few patients who simply didn't get nauseous from the potent drugs he was receiving, but he never once threw-up during the months of his intravenous chemotherapy. About an hour before he was to receive the IV infusion, I would give him some medications from a recipe all my own. Unfortunately I can no longer remember it entirely but it had acetaminophen, a fair number of different drugs in the Valium family, as well as compazine (a first-line nausea suppressant) and a bit of anti-histamine. It's true he could remember little of those Thursdays for medications in the diazepam family are well-known to produce anterograde amnesia. But the fact that Jack never experienced one sustained bout of nausea remains one of my most gratifying successes. Afterwards, as we drove home, Jack would doze in the car. Towards the end of his life he'd need help walking from the garage to our condo, but once there the exhausting chemotherapy would combine with my recipe and he would crawl into bed and fall fast asleep, his face relaxed, his body finally at rest.

As he became more ill and slept through Thursday nights, those hours after chemotherapy became my own, my one night when I could go out as Jack slept soundly. I once overheard Fred Lawrence talking to a straight friend about a gay couple, Bradly and Tom, the latter being in intensive care for prolonged periods. During the day, Bradly would be with Tom constantly. But at night, while his partner slept, Bradly would make his own rounds, going to bars and baths. The friend, hearing this, complained about Bradly's "infidelities." Fred's response was quick and unequivocal: he pointed out Bradly's devotion to Tom, his constant presence at the bedside while his partner was awake, his persistent loyalty throughout the long and draining illness. Who was to judge this person or his ethics? Such perspective could have applied to me—my Thursday nights could also have been condemned—for as Jack slept deeply those nights, I would take a few hours for myself. I spent my time in bars, drinking, socializing and diving into AIDS fund-raisers. For caregivers, time away is vital—for an army cannot fight without clothing, food, and rest.

Besides my Thursday night escapes, I found books to be reassuring. Reading medical journals was a necessity which left me without the spare time or focus to read novels or other books of length. But economy of words made poetry and plays accessible: I read, among others, John Donne, W. H. Auden, Thom Gunn, the plays of Tennessee Williams and Henrik Ibsen and "coffee table" books of the architecture of Frank Lloyd Wright and the Wiener Werkstätte design movement. When we traveled to Europe in 1989, I lugged along a far-too-heavy volume of my favorite poet, Edna St. Vincent Millay. I do not fit so readily into the e-society of today as I find a book's physicality is part of its appeal: the sturdiness of books promise survival in the face of inconstant electronics. Something in life, my books told me, evaded annihilation. But books and bars weren't my only escape. Every Sunday night there was a Rhythm & Blues TV program which drew my attention and anticipation. Music, also, provided solace in demonstrating the permanence of auditory pleasure when it seemed there were few other things left to enjoy. Music sang of the stability of ongoing life and reminded me that I was still alive and capable of responding! Books, bars and blues. These were a few comforts in a brutal routine.

THE TRIP-WIRE OF TEARS

Jack was never much of a tea drinker, but over the course of his treatment, his tastes changed and he began drinking tea. UCLA hospital couldn't necessarily give its patients longer lives, but it could provide them an extravagant selection of teas. Towards the end of his life now, he looked pale, gaunt and frail; he was weak and irritable and his impatience frazzled our bond. But every time I saw him in those days, my heart was scratched with the realization that he would soon be gone. How would I live without him? I am an introvert by nature, an extrovert by necessity; being around people drains me of energy, being alone charges my batteries. That is not to say that I, and other introverts, cannot rise to the occasion and be great successes at a party. But life is easier for an introvert when they can push an extrovert partner forward to "do the heavy lifting."

On a particularly frustrating day, Jack didn't like his tea which he blamed on me as I was serving as tea barista. We walked into the suite, more slowly than we ever had before, and once Jack was seated I traveled to its other end where the refreshments were. I had prepared his tea according to his specific instructions which were, I thought, maddeningly idiosyncratic and needlessly stringent. Perhaps he was exercising the only control he had, but my concoction was refused four times that day. Seeing Jack in that condition, however, defused any impatience or frustration I might have had. I was much aware that there, but for the grace of god, go I. This was not as hypothetical as it may seem: I was constantly aware that the virus was eating away at my immune system and could turn in a heartbeat and leave me with the same malignancy. It's easier to walk in someone else's shoes when your own instep is being measured.

As I was walking back and forth to the "Refreshment and Welcoming" counter, another nurse, who wasn't Jack's, noticed my meticulous preparation of his tea. She came to me, as I was pouring the hot water, and told me that Jack could not have had a better partner. It's an odd phenomenon—under great emotional stress we can plow along with whatever task we're given and we carefully hold our emotions in check until, often by accident, the beauty of our actions are recognized and an unseen psychological trip-wire is snagged. For me that day all the frustration and grief were released and I broke down sobbing. I don't recall the particular nurse's name, I may have never known it, but she knew mine.

DOUBLE TRAGEDY—
GEORGE KRIVACEK AND LLOYD BURR

Lloyd Burr eventually got a police "ankle bracelet" as a result of a DUI or some liquor store altercation—it was never clear which. In any case, he was confined to the house as a measure of public safety and George had to be the one to buy Lloyd liquor as he was the only one able to leave their house. At several points through the years, George had threatened breaking their relationship if Lloyd wouldn't stop drinking. Finally George had refused to buy any more alcohol—leaving Lloyd at home to navigate as best he could. Under the strain of being HIV-positive and cut off from liquor, Lloyd had taken a shotgun and fired it at his head. He'd done it in the living room of their home—only a few feet from where those dinners with the four of us had taken place. The county coroner had just left the house with Lloyd's body, George spoke in shock. Would I come over and help him clean up?

Looking back now it seems horribly absurd for the two of us to be cleaning up the blood, hair and bits of body tissue which remained. I simply didn't know one could hire professionals who are trained for such things as this. Upon arriving at the house and finding the inconceivably horrendous remains of human despair, I know I offered to clean up everything alone, without George's ashen-faced help. I should have insisted that he leave while I dealt with the scene of horror. But it was a time when many of us found ourselves doing things we never imagined.

But as I look back, there was a sacredness to our cleaning: a piety, a devotion, perhaps a penance, in our quiet work that day and well into the night. Also a farewell, far more prolonged than funerals provide, for those of us remaining on this planet. We are so different, one from another, in spite of our similar anatomy and circuitry, that I am sometimes amazed that we can understand each other at all. That it's even possible that we can speak the same language. And in this unknowable difference in finite and fragile muscle, bone and blood, who are we to judge our brothers? In that day, in that time, we took care of each other, buried each other and mourned each other. In the onslaught of so many deaths, the social conventions normally guiding us were irrelevant. Each of us could be struck down at any minute, as if by gunfire, as if in war, while society functioned normally around us. The San Francisco gay newspaper, *Bay Area Reporter*, filled two pages every Thursday with obituaries and we read in wonder and dread who had died the preceding week. The paper, early on, was forced to make strict rules for obituary submission in order to have enough space for them all. Meanwhile in the mainstream culture, news of our devastation remained minimized or absent. In such a world of imminent death and relentless loss, in this subculture of grief, we made our own rules and rituals of death as best we could. It was in this spirit of not knowing the unknowable in the human kneeling beside me that I didn't push George to let me do the whole clean-up job by myself.

* * *

It was during the last month of my practice that George Krivacek came to me with a vial of "Chinese Compound Q." The top of the vial wasn't capped in a sterile manner and I asked him what he wanted me to do with the amber liquid.

"Inject it into me."

"George, to start with, it's not a sterile solution in a sterile vial. Secondly, we don't know what it is and we have no idea what it will actually do."

"It's doing amazing things according to underground druggies. Some say it's a cure that the U.S. government just doesn't want us to have," he replied.

"Ah, George, we've been over this. There's no one in the U.S. government smart enough to come up with HIV. And there's nothing they don't want you to have; if anything, they don't care about you."

"Andrew, you know I love you, but you can be very naïve about the government and what it's doing." He threatened to inject it himself at home, alone, in non-sterile conditions. He believed Compound Q was a wonder drug, but he preferred to have me there. He trusted me, he said. George was unshakeable.

It was with a heavy heart that I took the vial and irradiated it at our hospital. I knew there was no way I could inject him there; I had the hospital's legal standing to protect as well as my license. Looking back, at the least I should have had a chemical analysis performed. If I refused him, would he really inject himself? We went to his house in the Valley, just the two of us. I entreated him again not to go through with it. Although AZT had sickened him beyond tolerance and he'd stopped it, his health didn't seem to be declining. But now I echoed my Intensive Care Attendings: who knew when a cure would be discovered? It could be tomorrow, I said. He waved away such a possibility.

"If we're going to do it, and we are, let's do it," he said.

He lay down on the living room couch, with Lloyd's blood still staining the floor beneath us, steps away from the dining table where the four of us had eaten. He lay back. I filled the syringe from the vial and prepared his arm.

"One last chance, George, to say no. We don't know what this is."

"Just do it."

It was to be one of the greatest mistakes of my life.

I planted the needle and injected the yellowish fluid. Within a few minutes he blanched and threw up. I dialed 911.

George Krivacek was never the same. His unconsciousness in the first few hours grew into an agitated coma—a condition that can appear to an onlooker as if the individual is having horrible nightmares but cannot awaken. After nearly two weeks of intensive care, he finally awoke. Horribly gaunt when he was discharged a few weeks later, the sparkle had left his eyes.

I heard of his passing in some off-the-cuff remark by a mutual friend a few months later. And so it went. Later, after Jack's death, I'd be out at a bar and meet some friend of a patient, or a friend of someone I knew. Perhaps an intelligent or witty guy, someone fun and lively. Someone who could help lift me out of the morass of sadness and shut out the future I believed was waiting for me. Maybe we'd have a couple of beers together and share bits of our lives, but we'd carefully avoid any mention of AIDS, or sickness, or death. We'd exchange phone numbers or maybe not. And then in a couple months or so, I'd run into him. "Hey, what's Mike, or Tom, or Jim doing?" I'd ask. "Oh, he died two weeks ago," I'd hear in reply—referring to our mutual friend. By that time, we wouldn't say things like "Sorry to tell you" or "Didn't you know?" It was just a fact. One of many ordinary facts. One of many deaths.

DON WHITMAN

I saw Don Whitman for the first time in our offices on a Friday when he needed immediate hospitalization. He was slightly short of breath, coughing frequently, and on his lower chest exam I could hear constricted airways in both lungs. He was thin, but hadn't yet reached the point of obvious emaciation. He displayed the hallmark seborrheic dermatitis between his eyes, on his forehead, in the creases around his nose. After this initial evaluation I admitted him to the hospital and started him on pentamidine even before his chest X-ray results were known.

When I next saw him he was on an oxygen mask and each of his arms had an IV line—one with pentamidine to fight his pneumonia and one for access and fluids. I asked him how he was doing and he replied that he was fine. While I puzzled over how to start the conversation, and whether his psyche could accept the information at that moment, he spoke again. It was difficult to hear him over the hiss of the oxygen mask and the beeps of his finger oximeter. I leaned closer, now above him.

"What did you say, Don?"

"I need..." he spoke through his breathlessness. "I need to be back at work on Monday."

The cognitive dissonance was striking. It was Friday and it was doubtful he would last a week. But his question informed me that, in spite of the objective clarity of his situation, he didn't understand what little time he had.

"Don," I started—but we were interrupted by the entrance of a nurse and a nurse's aid bringing him a meal he couldn't eat.

"Excuse me," I said, "we need a little time here." The irony of my words ricocheted in my head, behind my glasses. My eyes stayed on him as they left the room. "Don, you're very, very sick. You are dying. Do you have a partner or some close friends you can call to be with you?" I asked.

"Yes," he spoke between breaths, "I've got a buddy in West Hollywood and my sister is in Denver."

"You should call them right away because you need help."

Although his oxygen saturation fell through the night and into the next day, and I told him his life would soon be over, he didn't agree to "Do Not Resuscitate" orders. But he had called his friend and sister.

Years later my physician Mark Higgins, M.D., taught me that, as a routine part of a complete assessment, he asked every patient how many friends he or she had that were HIV-positive or had passed away. In order to understand a patient's all-important expectations, it is vital to know the extent of their acquaintance with people with AIDS—and therefore the course of the disease itself. Evidently Don knew few, if any, people who had AIDS.

Don barely survived the weekend. He died Monday after a futile resuscitation attempt by the doctor on staff and nurses with the "crash cart." He had stepped off the earth only three days after his hospital admission.

LAST YEAR OF PRACTICE

About a year before I left the practice, Fred Lawrence hired two accomplished, published neurologists, one being Elaine Feraru, M.D. Shortly before disability forced me to leave LMG, the other neurologist resigned. Although his departure didn't affect me directly, it added a bit of uncertainty and instability to our office precisely when things were growing more difficult and unsteady for me. It was at this point Fred asked me to increase my hospital in-patient responsibilities which meant dealing with more end-of-life issues than what was routinely found in our clinic.

It had become apparent that I had a gift for assisting the dying. While I could lessen the universal fear of pain at the end of a person's life and perhaps help mend a broken relationship, I found I was able to provide substantially more. The most important thing a physician can create, whether dealing with a terminal illness or not, is connectedness. Physical presence alone, which was all I was sometimes allowed, produces powerful connection. But even more than that, I could connect with my patients by listening—not talking but simply listening. While my own personal HIV diagnosis was unspoken, I always felt its silent presence and it magnified my ability to connect. In their triumph or despair, I could stand where my patients stood. And I have no doubt that the people I served could feel this resonance. While I couldn't provide a cure, I could be present and listen attentively. I could battle isolation of the soul.

In helping those dying reach some relief in the last days or weeks of their lives, my work was appreciated not only by LMG, but also by physicians outside the group. Often unsure of optimum HIV care and uncomfortable with end-of-life issues, it wasn't unusual for doctors

ANDREW M. FAULK, M.D.

to transfer patients to the care of LMG. It is without exaggeration to say that Vincent, Fred and other LMG physicians could hospitalize their patients under my care without concern—either for correct technical diligence or for psychological attention.

During the years of my practice, I found several suggestions I recommend to friends and loved ones of the dying to help gain some closure during their last conversations:

1) I love you.
2) Please forgive me for whatever disappointment or offense I have caused (even if you believe the dying person was at fault—it's only your ego, not your life.)
3) I forgive you for the disappointments or offenses you have caused.
4) Thank you for your part in my life.
5) I will miss you.
6) Perhaps review with the dying person some important fun, or funny, shared event, circumstance, or person, and, finally,
7) Good-bye.

So during the last months of my practice, I was assigned more hospital rounds and proportionally less office practice. Hospitalized patients are sicker, of course, and while I didn't mind expanding the technical side of care, their intense emotional demands began to take a toll on me. Lawrence Medical was truly accommodating in giving me every Thursday off in order to accompany Jack to chemotherapy at UCLA, and did so without complaint. But at that point caring for additional hospitalized patients was an emotional drain I could ill afford. I had given my ear and heart as best I could, but with some cost to myself. I had gone to three Goodbye Parties and one funeral in three years and I was learning that grief is cumulative; the death of even the least-known patient, transferred to me just hours before his demise, had weight. By postponing grief's full expression, I was only papering over what I would feel much more painfully later.

I began to forget the names of well-known patients. When on-call I had difficulty identifying the crux of patients' complaints. In order to jog my memory, I began to take home the charts of patients likely to call. I was losing sense of exactly when I had ordered what medication—especially those prescriptions I had phoned into the hospital or local pharmacies. The dosages of common medications began to slip my mind and I even began to lose that subconscious knowledge of which day of the week it is.

I was forgetting too much.

And then Fred Lawrence became ill. Due to the legal reasons I've described, we physicians did not inquire as to each other's HIV status. I didn't know that of other LMG doctors and they didn't know mine. Fred had begun practice in the relatively innocent days of mere STDs: gonorrhea, syphilis, non-specific urethritis, etc. When HIV emerged he rode the swell, as I did, of medical need. He was never board certified in Family Practice, choosing instead to exit academia sooner rather than later and trust his own capabilities and entrepreneurial instincts. He had made the switch from easy, cookbook medicine to the obscure nuances and harsh realities of what was then one of the least understood diseases in medicine. And he had made the transition with flying colors. Now he himself was ill.

Our neurologist Elaine came to me in the Immunosuppression Unit of North Hollywood's community hospital. I was taken aback when she took me into a small nursing supply room and closed the door. As she sought such privacy, I assumed yet another of the doctors or office staff had become ill or, in that brutal world of the 1980s and '90s, been found dead. It was the former, but the physician was Dr. Lawrence himself.

The space was small—it hadn't been designed to house people.

"Fred's sick," she said. "His chest X-ray is whited out." I was caught off-guard. Even though we were living in a world where death was a constant occurrence, my surprise was proportional to his emotional proximity.

"How long has he been sick?" I asked.

"He's had a non-productive cough for ten days, maybe two weeks," Elaine answered. "I need your help," she continued. "He refuses to come into the hospital. You know Fred, he insists on being treated at home."

I slowly digested the shock. He was a gay man active during the worst years of contagion and his illness should not have been a great surprise. But he was a doctor, and our training had taught us that, as physicians, we were indestructible. We didn't become sick. We had gone through a training which involved years of astonishing amounts of work and sleep deprivation. Our responsibilities and schedules were such that anything approaching illness was simply not acknowledged. Although we had freely chosen our grueling work, if some of us obnoxiously considered ourselves gods, it was because the superhuman had been expected of us. And we had often risen to the challenge. However such convictions were as much myth as was Fred's health and immortality. His X-ray was snowing lethal white. He had *Pneumocystis* pneumonia.

The enemy was at the gate.

Fred's bed was a huge affair with an enormous canopy from which Elaine had initially hung the bags of pentamidine before an IV pole had arrived. As he felt comfortable with her, only once did I make the drive over to his house in the Hollywood Hills to hang a bag. But the shock of his illness was as profound as if I had diagnosed the infection in a lover; in the office, we'd already lost some of our staff. At home I was navigating the tortuous paths of Jack's medical schedules and his roller coaster of emotions while my hospital workload was increasingly weighted towards the sickest. Before Fred's diagnosis I had requested that I do less hospital work but with the loss of Dr. Olson and the other neurologist I was told that working less wasn't possible. I was seeing more hospitalized patients.

MY LAST DAY IN PRACTICE

It had been a full week with a good number of patients in the hospital, many quite ill with three, in particular, who would certainly not survive longer than a few days. There had been a family conference scheduled for one of them. Work was increasingly demanding as my mind was clouded and I required extra effort to remember the details of those drugs we, in fact, used frequently. I was preoccupied with the death of our colleague Luke Olson, and the increase in work from his and Fred's absence had put Vincent, as well as the office staff, on edge.

While Jack's energy and mood rose and fell from day to day, his chemotherapy treatment had been a particular challenge. He hadn't experienced nausea or vomiting, but those mere possibilities paled in contrast to the actualities of those present. The body aches, headaches and overwhelming fatigue—the general discomfort— were beginning to weigh on him. Although I hadn't noticed evidence per se, I was beginning to feel that he and I were drifting apart as his illness began to take up more of his energies and attention. There was less enthusiasm as I walked in the door each night, fewer of his manufactured pratfalls; music and TV shows became more irritating than distracting as he sought the comfort of sleep.

It was a Saturday and the day was to be a full one. After rounding on hospitalized patients, I had a day of appointments waiting for me at the Wilshire office. Elaine was also seeing patients that day and she had asked me to go out to dinner with her that night.

Meanwhile I just wanted to lie down.

At the hospital, I reviewed my first patient's chart and then examined him. He was young, somewhere in his late 20s. Whatever

ANDREW M. FAULK, M.D.

his diagnoses were, John wasn't going to survive long and his family needed to be told. The family was soon gathered in one of the conference rooms and as I told them of his imminent death, to my consternation I began to tear. I felt distant, emotionally detached, as if I were outside my body watching myself. My tears fell down my cheeks obscuring the chart. The family was grief-stricken over their son's approaching death but, it was easy to see, further confused and, I imagine, dismayed by their doctor's tears.

There are times when it's not necessarily bad for one's physician to cry. But this hadn't been one of those times; I had needed to be strong and confident and I hadn't been.

To worsen the situation, I hadn't remembered that there were two more family conferences scheduled in which each family needed to be told that it was unlikely their son and brother would survive more than a few days. Each time I cried and each time it was inappropriate. I couldn't remember when I'd lost my composure this way. What was happening?

TO WORK, OR TO LIVE

Although Elaine was wearing down my resistance, I continued to refuse dinner with her. I was bewildered over what had happened that morning—that and the fatigue of the day was at the heart of my refusal. I was feeling overwhelmed but simultaneously, without fully realizing it, oddly distanced. She must have seen the desperation just beneath the surface, for she wouldn't accept my refusal.

Over the course of dinner, I became the object of our mutual attention; I confessed my exhaustion and I reviewed the disturbing tears I had experienced at that morning's family meetings. Together we reviewed the trouble I was having remembering simple medications. I disclosed that I was HIV-positive—something I had never divulged to any physician with whom I was working. Elaine did not stay quiet: she interrupted several times to ask for pertinent details. How was I managing Jack and his malignancy? She was listening as a sympathetic friend, but she was also collecting data as a trained neurologist who specialized in HIV.

After considering the information she shocked me to my core, "You've got to quit."

What? She couldn't be serious! I contested her opinion. I said I was just exhausted, somewhat depressed and at most needed some time off. But in a few moments the hard realization hit me—*I had secretly been wishing I would contract pneumonia.* If I were ill, I could at last escape what had become a terrible, crushing burden. Tears of that morning became tears of that night.

"If you want to get sick, this is a disease that will give you what you wish for," she responded. "the practice will survive without you."

ANDREW M. FAULK, M.D.

She was resolute. "Right now. Absolutely. You can't go back to work."

There were sirens in my head. I couldn't breathe.

Elaine was as wise as she was dispassionate. She was doing her job; it was a speech the both of us had given many times before. But this time I wasn't giving it, I was the one hearing it.

Usually a job is necessary to earn a living and, if one is fortunate, engage our minds and passions as it consumes our time. But for some a job is experienced as identity. For my physical and emotional health, to attain an untroubled, low-stress life, Elaine was voicing the unthinkable: I needed to leave this definition of myself behind. So it was during that dinner in a Studio City restaurant that it all came crashing down around my ears. For the second time in my life, I fought a battle to keep my profession. Although she thought there was a chance it was merely depression, she was doubtful. Just as before, this was a choice between preserving my career or preserving my health.

The sirens in my head went silent. The world stopped. I knew in that shattering instant that she was right. My survival trumped everything: freshman chemistry with the T.A. who spoke no English, the barely-managed terror of Organic Chemistry, the essays on political discourse, the hours of research, the mind-snapping tests, numberless discussions with professors, Attendings, study groups; diligent patient examinations; the punishing enforced sleep deprivation of scores of on-call nights. Their hard-fought result was now to be relinquished.

Elaine had said it all: "If you want to be sick, this is a disease which will give you what you wish for." It was Saturday—I called Vincent and the wheels of my future began to realign.

As long as I had thought that my difficulties might be attributable to depression, I had something of a cushion from imagining my career was ended. While some HIV dementia was certainly possible, I held on to the hope my memory problems were due to simple depression. Neurologic testing in the days ahead would show that the source wasn't depression, but rather HIV encephalopathy—HIV impacting the functions of the brain. My career was over. But my life was not.

RESIGNING FROM
LAWRENCE MEDICAL GROUP

So it was in February of 1991 that my departure from medicine came. Jack was into month five of his chemotherapy at UCLA. I was caring for more and more hospitalized patients, and many of the most psychologically distressed were being transferred to my care. Luke Olson, M.D., had been hospitalized and passed away the November before. Fred had just recovered from his own bout with PCP. And then there were the deaths of other Lawrence Medical staff; we had lost Mark our office assistant the preceding fall and another office assistant—before he had been there long enough for me to learn his name—had been found dead in his car off the I-405. We were now losing about two patients per week to the disease. My discussion with Elaine had occurred two days before. It was time.

> To All My Patients,
> Effective February 4, 1991, I am taking an indefinite leave of absence from my responsibilities here at Lawrence Medical Group. In order to meet some challenges at home, and remain available for the future needs of our community, I am withdrawing from the practice for the time being. This has not been a particularly easy decision, but as I am sure one can readily understand, we are involved in a special work which occasionally requires special considerations. A great comfort to me is the knowledge that the care you receive here at Lawrence Medical is unsurpassed, unsurpassed not only in the sense of up-to-the-minute technical sophistication, but also unsurpassed in the sense of providing this care in

　　　　　ANDREW M. FAULK, M.D.

the context of human dignity and with the understanding of the paramount importance of the quality of life.

This context of care is an understanding of priorities which is identical to that which has always been my personal and professional goal.

I remain available to help smooth whatever difficulties this transition may represent for you and thank you, in advance, for your understanding and support. I will miss you all.

Sincerely Yours,
Andrew M. Faulk, M.D.

DEPARTURE FROM PRACTICE

My departure from medicine and the career I loved is a difficult story to tell. As an undergraduate at Columbia, I double-majored in pre-medicine and political science. I couldn't really know what a career in medicine would mean and I certainly didn't comprehend the time and sacrifices required but I did know the long march through medical school, internship and residency required years. I was a pauper while my graduated friends had jobs and incomes and girlfriends/boyfriends/spouses and children. Without these I felt like an adolescent, my social life had been frozen in time. I had had no time and no money and I felt it.

After graduation from college, while waiting for medical school, my work at the law firm of White & Case had given me a regular job where I saw a disturbing distillation of this profession. Those attorneys below the level of partner were demoralized and, to a person, passionately discouraged anyone from making law a career. Lawyers were fighters, it seemed; doctors were lovers. And my identity as the latter was certain—I was a nurturer. In medicine I was needed. In anything else I wondered that I wouldn't feel, and indeed be, superfluous.

With my identity intimately tied to my work, it has been a strain to separate the two. In fact, should you ask those who love me, they would tell you it's an enormous issue with which I still contend. My role in HIV medicine allowed me a first-hand look at the horror of the infection, the possibility of creeping dementia, and random sudden death. To contest my own doctors' judgment and stay in practice would have been unconscionable in light of the responsibility I had for my patients' care and safety. It was one of the most difficult moments of my life when I realized (after my departure from Lawrence Medical Group) that I'd never again be walking through the door of my office and seeing patients—my beloved guys, the children of Hamelin. I've had to surrender much of my identity as a physician and create anew from that which remains.

The advent of AIDS produced not just the waste of lives, as if anything more could matter, but also this loss of my profession—and with it a measure of my identity. These days, I'm most often aware of the forfeiture of my career when an acquaintance or friend discusses his or her symptoms, or a disease of some friend or relative, with didactic analysis of which symptom correlates with which disease (some people right, some wrong)—all showing that they have no awareness that I myself, standing there, am a physician. My training and experience are lost; my identity is mislaid.

I carry with me a weighted past (as does everyone): years of intensive study and sacrifice. But I don't regret these years, for I chose this road myself and others would have dearly loved the opportunities I've had. After all, I've had the supreme honor of being allowed to provide care for many of my brothers before they were taken from us—and for that I am deeply grateful.

SUNDAY ESCAPES TO THE GETTY

For the last year and a half of his life, Jack and I traveled to the Malibu Getty Museum for lunch most Sundays. Whether or not we went, I made reservations for every Sunday, my day off, in case he felt up to it. The Getty Villa was a recreation of a Roman nobleman's house, complete with enclosed patios with fountains and sitting areas surrounded by busts and extravagant depictions of Romans at work and play. From the acanthus leaves in the wall decorations (signifying long life) to the museum's most prized Van Gogh painting of sunflowers, Jack and I drank it all in. We would concentrate on just one room of the museum or quietly sit in one of its patios. At the museum we didn't need to talk, we just enjoyed each other's simple presence. This quiet reflection was all followed by a leisurely lunch outside in the sun under a latticework of vines and flowers. Jack and I spent many relaxing Sundays in those surroundings enjoyed by the aristocracy of ancient Rome.

We had discovered this relatively unknown jewel of Los Angeles long before his diagnosis of lymphoma and enjoyed it long after. On our last trip to the Getty, he had lost much of his hair and his weight had deteriorated, his cheeks were sunken, his skin tawny beyond natural. To his credit, he didn't complain during his decline. When he had enjoyed what he had the energy for, he would merely ask "Why don't we go?" With each visit, more and more slowly, we'd walk back down to the car together and head home for the remainder of a sleepy Sunday.

LINGERING REGRETS

In the beginning, Jack was able to maintain a matter-of-factness about his malignancy. But as his illness progressed and it became clear chemotherapy was ineffective, grief overcame him and tangled his emotions. During his last months, facing his inevitable death, I sometimes became a target of his frustration. Anger at caregivers is common, I have seen couples break up when the patient had only a few months to live (or sudden romances begun with equally abbreviated life spans). While I'm sadly familiar with the phenomenon, the sting was hard to take.

About three months before he died, Jack overheard my end of a telephone conversation which upset him tremendously. I had been downstairs in the kitchen while he lay in bed upstairs. I can no longer remember with whom I was speaking, but the question came up concerning how long he was expected to live. "A few months," I replied with a remote, professional matter-of-factness behind which I would occasionally hide. Unfortunately Jack overheard my half of the conversation and was bowled over by what he heard to be the definitive prognosis and, in addition, he interpreted my remarks as a wish rather than a report. When I saw his agony, I tried to convince him that my statement had nothing to do with desire, but the prediction was more difficult to discount. I told him that I happily imagined his presence with me long into the future. But by that time the fatigue and pain he felt, the tedium of sickness, the frustrated wishes of a life un-lived: all of these worked his emotions into a state in which they imploded into an uncharacteristic paranoia. My remarks left him despairing and bitter and my efforts in explanation, sadly, fell flat and disbelieved. He remained angry with me, on and off, until he passed away. This was to be a great sorrow of my life, that during the last few months of his life there was tension between us. But perhaps his reaction to this overheard phone call was a sign that his illness had finally bested him. If so, I cannot blame him.

JACK'S RIGHT TO LAST RITES

Throughout the years of my practice, I submerged my personal spiritual beliefs in order to provide the most support possible for my patients. Part of my work was to protect each individual's own personal faith, without exhibiting a zeal for their faith which would have looked as phony as it would have been. Had I had such believer's consolation, my life and work would have been easier. But my upbringing in the church has inoculated me, as it were, from religion: religious belief, it seems, can't be organic in me. Even if my patient's near-death experience wasn't due to undiscovered human communication and signals from a dying brain, an afterlife seems implausible. In any case, this is a cognitive dissonance I can't resolve. All those in my care deserved whatever religious attention they desired; if I could not provide it, I would facilitate their getting it elsewhere. Jack was to receive no less.

For as long as I knew him, he had never attended Mass. Nevertheless, he considered himself a Catholic—not devout perhaps, but certainly within the Church. His Catholicism seemed to be more a piece of identity, a place for him in a social construct, rather than a rigid set of beliefs. Not being Catholic, the Evangelical teachings of my youth had always held this type of religious expression to be heretical. But regardless of doctrine he lived a life entirely consistent with a belief in God.

When we made that vacation to Europe in the fall of 1989, not knowing his reaction but wanting to be supportive, I floated the idea of visiting the Vatican and perhaps be in attendance at an appearance of the Pope. Would he see healing, or at least comfort, in the earthly embodiment of his faith? The first time I broached the topic, he paused a while before answering. Finally he said yes, but without great enthusiasm. Lourdes, it occurred to me suddenly, might be something he'd appreciate more and, who knew, perhaps it would better kindle a hope—hope, our most necessary of currencies—if not for healing, then for something else intangible. But he had no desire to make the journey to Lourdes. I searched for a papal schedule. This was Jack's life, after all, and I wasn't going to discourage him from any metaphysical comfort. Once we were in Rome, he became more interested in attending a papal display of whatever sort. As I suspected, he wasn't expecting any kind of cure, he only came searching for some bits of hope or comfort which even he couldn't define. But during our stay, contrary to his published schedule, Pope John Paul II stayed at his summer residence and didn't give any Vatican benedictions. Without a word of complaint or discouragement, Jack quietly settled for a papal medallion keychain and a resin angel which he hung above his bedpost at home.

Later, when his illness had progressed, I wrote my father asking for any Bible verses he could give that would be comforting and I could share with Jack. My father, with his vast knowledge of the Bible, could surely provide us with some moving pieces to console Jack in his last few weeks. My father, however, sent me "The 4 Spiritual Laws" Evangelical tract—a booklet used to convert non-believers. It was far from the warm and supporting scripture I had imagined. I didn't show it to Jack; I didn't think he needed another medallion keychain.

During his last hospitalization in May, 1991, it was clear he was not going to live much longer. I was distraught, unsure of what to say, what to do. Sickened by his cancer, his breathing became progressively labored. There came a moment, an hour, when it appeared that he was failing. Not knowing what "Extreme Unction" or "Last Rites" actually involved, but believing it an integral part of Catholicism, I was going to do all I could for Jack to participate in it while he was sufficiently aware. He wanted it—that was all that was necessary. Not knowing who would step off the earth first, we had made a commitment to support each other as best we could. His hour of death may have been uncertain, but he had chosen this sacrament of the Church, and to be cognizant during it.

That afternoon at UCLA Hospital, I called the hospital chaplain and requested "Extreme Unction" (also known as the "Sacrament of the Sick" and therefore not limited to those who are dying). After some three hours, a priest was found. I had started the process before Jack's mother Viv returned from a break because I knew, for whatever reason, she would be in opposition. Once she learned of my efforts to procure a priest, she was livid—she demanded the ceremony be stopped. Perhaps it wasn't my decision she resented, perhaps she believed he would be shaken if he knew we thought he was failing. That was possibly true, although I found it an unsettling testament to her faith that she believed the "Sacrament of the Sick" would be more demoralizing than comforting. Subsequent research has shown, however, that a patient's understanding of his or her illness doesn't rob them of hope and calm but, besides providing these essential elements, decreases terror, worry and depression. It also gives him and his family and loved ones time to prepare emotionally and logistically for what is to come. In any case Jack had been adamant that he would receive all of the Church's rites. Viv could storm into the room and throw her opinions and orders around, but she could not countermand his choices made in quieter moments. If he wanted "Extreme Unction" I would see he got it.

He received this sacrament and was, as I had hoped, conscious enough to participate. But he did live to go home once more and I saw that Viv felt vindicated. My mind was numb, my emotions raw: it is impossible for me to say what I felt during those hours between his hospital discharge and his death. I'm sure triumph was not the only sentiment Viv had and perhaps I misread her. But this is how it appeared.

PERMANENT LOSS

Jack died in the living room of our condominium, in front of the wet bar, in a hospital bed we had rented the week before. Three days prior, he had been discharged from the UCLA Medical Center with hospice care being our only option. The day before he died, in a voice which was hardly more than a whisper, he asked what would be done next—not what could be done, but what would be done. Even hours before his death, Jack, like all of us, needed hope. I told him a fantasy, cloaked in medical jargon, of some remaining treatment. There was still hope, I lied.

But many others were like him; they weren't ready to be told that death was near. Don, the hard-working attorney, on his Friday hospital admission, told me he needed to return to work Monday. His 6'1" frame weighed no more than 100 pounds when I told him that we would do our best. As always, I was to take my cues from the patient, for there is no right way or wrong way to die. This time it was my Jack. If someone wasn't ready for death, it wasn't my place to drag them, kicking and screaming, to a point of accepting something which they couldn't.

Ominously, he had stopped clucking altogether.

I stayed with him on and off through those nights, sometimes sleeping upstairs in our bedroom but usually napping with my head on his bed. I wandered outside from time to time to watch the ripples on the pool outside our door. I've never been a smoker, but I wished I had been in order to gain whatever smokers gain. I wanted him to live forever, and I wanted him to die in the next hour. I wanted him back the way he had always been.

It was in the morning hours of June 4, 1991, when Jack finally

ANDREW M. FAULK, M.D.

passed away, at the age of 43. Over the course of those eight months after his lymphoma diagnosis he had lost 30 pounds and his sparkling smile, but not his will to live. He never gave up and in that there is its own triumph. Denial on the part of one who is dying, or his loved ones, may well impede a tranquility that acceptance would supply but there is something to be said for a durable hope, for an optimism in the face of constant deterioration and accelerating loss.

Over those last weeks with Jack, I had a recurrent image, a mirage, that lingered on the edge of my consciousness, and which reflected the last steps of the journey we made together. In the daydream I am carrying a sleeping Jack in my arms. He is quiet and peaceful, no longer in pain or fear, and I am able to carry him easily—his weight is not a burden. This half-dream gave me a strange and difficult-to-describe solace.

JACK'S DEATH AND OUR MARRIAGE RING

During those dark days of chemotherapy, after he had lost too much hair and too many pounds, we found ourselves sitting in a little Orange Julius in a nearby shopping mall. It was there that Jack asked if I wouldn't on occasion wear his ring. To this day it pains me deeply to think he needed to ask for something that was to happen naturally and with reverence. I told him absolutely yes, and there before me, as he sat gaunt and grey-colored, I saw again the smile I had seen on his face those years back in Venice.

There are few things I remember clearly from that morning he died but the most vivid memory I have is of my quickly taking off his precious ring after his breathing stopped and his eyes glazed. Before it was lost or, more likely, confiscated by his mother. Viv had done an inventory of our house during the preceding week and it was clear she intended to take everything she could: everything that Jack owned before he met me, everything we acquired together and anything else she could. And if, in her espionage, she couldn't ascertain what was mine and what was ours, she wouldn't be splitting hairs; if in doubt, I knew, she intended to take what she could carry. The moments immediately after he passed, my objective was uncomplicated— through my tears I slipped the ring off his fourth finger and put it on my own. Jack would get his wish: I would wear his ring, our ring, and he would be remembered, and cherished in that remembrance.

When the two EMT men arrived to take his body away, they asked me if I wouldn't rather step out of the room while they placed him in the body-bag. I said no, I wasn't going to leave him. I sat while they put on plastic gloves and gingerly lifted his corpse, still warm, from the bed and placed his still form in the large black bag

ANDREW M. FAULK, M.D.

and zipped it shut. As is part of our humanity, we feel there is still a part of the person we knew in their remains. For so there is. We honor those bodies of the ones we love. We carefully bury them. We visit their graves. It was only when the EMT men insisted that I not ride along to the mortuary, that it was against their rules, it was only then that I acquiesced and let his body go.

JACK'S FUNERAL AND
THE BRUTAL AFTERMATH

Our office manager Pam came to my rescue. She began calling those who needed to know and she arranged for a funeral Mass in a nearby Catholic church. Although I had anticipated dealing with the funeral home, I was grateful when Pam began the planning for me. During Jack's last hospitalization, he was so close to death that I had asked him whether he preferred cremation or burial and, if internment, where. When we first moved to Los Angeles, we had gone on a light-hearted tour of celebrities' grave sites. The sinking realization of what we both faced, however, soon twisted the tour into something far more serious than when begun. But neither of us had had anything definitive to say on our burial preference. Now at a far more serious time I was asking where would he like to be buried. "Well, where are *you* going to be buried?" he asked. "I don't know, Jack, but whatever may happen in my life, even if I might have another relationship, I will be buried with you."

In the end he couldn't decide; he was just too sick to choose a location for his grave. In looking back, I am troubled by my persistence that day—in spite of our previous discussions, I was asking too much of him. The time for such decisions had passed. After all, legally I was little more than a roommate. Viv and Gus stepped into the vacuum and, over Pam's objections and my peripheral input—domestic partnership, let alone marriage, was not even a dream at that time—the funeral home gave his parents sole control of his burial. Without discussion or debate, Jack was buried in Collinsville, Illinois. Had it been another time, or had I been another man, I would have

ANDREW M. FAULK, M.D.

demanded I be included in, if not directing, the planning. But I had neither instructions from Jack nor the energy to battle his parents.

Viv vociferously fought against any ceremony—either a funeral or a memorial—in California or back in Illinois. He had insisted that there be no viewing of his body, but he had definitely wanted a funeral Mass. She was beginning to chip away at what I knew he had wanted. There were many, many who had known this wonderful, sweet man and they deserved the opportunity to honor him, to say goodbye at some type of service. I overruled her: there would be a Mass. If there were to be a Mass, she declared, then at least there were to be no flowers. I was shocked—Jack had been a sometime florist! No, I insisted, there were going to be flowers. If there were to be flowers, she persisted, then there was to be no music. What? Was she kidding? Flowers and music at a funeral or memorial service were so universal that it was absurd to oppose them. I was dumbstruck! If she had her way there would be no Mass, no flowers, no music! She disliked me intensely and that could be sufficient fuel for disagreement but it seems unbelievable she would reject or minimize any formal ceremony just to prove superior power. It seemed like it was partially due to a problem with Jack—perhaps it was anger, perhaps shame with him for his sexual orientation—I can only speculate as to her motives. Powered or not by her challenge from me or her disgust with Jack, I found her remonstrations to be absurd and heartless. This painfully showed me just how far issues of power and control can hijack common tradition and common sense.

Now I fought her not as a powerless roommate but as his spouse. There would be all three—a Mass, music and flowers. I was determined. My plans and resolve, however, thwarted her into full fury.

"Let's get on with it. I just want to get him into the ground as fast as possible so I can get on with my life."

How could anyone feel that way about playful, loving Jack? How could anyone say that? I was stunned to the core. Sadly, Viv's attitude was not hers alone. Years before a mother had asked me, while her 23-year-old son lay dying in the Intensive Care Unit, exactly when he would die because she needed to get back East for work. That mother had said the same thing as Viv: "Just get him buried."

Viv and Gus ignored the physical care and emotional support Jack received from me; this was the attitude of many families toward the partners and boyfriends who provided such loving care during those dark days. We caregivers often worked alone and without acknowledgment. The months I cared for him, I had changed soiled sheets, run for a bedpan, searched for that one food he liked and might eat. I had spent time taking him to doctors' appointments, sitting with him during chemotherapy and those small hours of the night when the terror of approaching death demanded alliance and understanding. Like so many of my brothers, I made the sacrifice of complete submersion in the life of a dying man to the neglect of my own. But once Jack was gone, once our brothers had passed, we caregivers were frequently left with no notice of our efforts and no one to share our loss.

The funeral Mass was conducted in a Catholic church not far from where we lived, by a priest who had never known him. Although the priest forgot to call me up to the podium for my eulogy—a poem of mine that had written itself—the organist remembered my song request, John Lennon's "Imagine." Outside the church the sunlight was blinding. I don't know if Gus and Viv were there; I have no memory of them. The Soehlke's and I did not grieve together.

I didn't mind as Viv and Gus began taking items from the house. I noticed absent-mindedly that they evidently had no plans for taking the furniture—for which I was glad. The condo and its furnishings, I thought, were some of the few things that still tied me to Jack. However my mind pivoted—many ancient civilizations took the deceased's earthly possessions and either buried them, or burned them, along with the body. Jack was gone. Did it matter what physical expressions remained? Suddenly, it seemed, removing many of his contributions to our life was not as awful as it first appeared. Now it hardly mattered what they took—I would have his memory. During this pillaging of the house, standing in the kitchen I nevertheless mentioned some item I wanted to keep.

Viv turned on me. "Don't you get it? You dumb son of a bitch!" Back in our office there was much free-floating anger, but an unbreakable rule of the practice was that no one was allowed to call the staff or doctors names.

"Why are you alive? Why are you still alive when you gave it to him? Answer me that, big AIDS doctor, *why are you still alive when he's dead*?"

My mind collapsed as my body stiffened. She was wrong on so

many levels. In fact I myself was facing no other end than that of my brothers, no different from that of my beloved Jack. After all, I was another son of Hamelin. I might have explained that her assumption was technically impossible. Jack had never been tested for HIV and without significant treatment available, it was not something I pressured him to do. Our sex life had always been conducted carefully. But the only thing I said was "That's not what happened. It didn't happen that way."

For the first time in many years, I wept. It all came out, the sobbing, the tears. Bleary-eyed I looked down at the kitchen counter and in that moment, for me, the entirety of Jack focused: his charm, his caring, his gentleness, his spirit. I didn't care that Viv saw me crying; I didn't care that she might interpret my tears as some kind of admission of guilt. Apparently the honesty in my voice and my tears communicated more than my lack of explanation.

"Well, if you didn't do it, one of you did. One of you sick perverts."

So it was finally out, the reason for all the anger, all the obstruction and bitterness I had always felt from her. Yes, I had seen disinterest in so many families for the caregivers. But this was different from the usual apathy. Viv had been angry since the day I met her and now she voiced her rage and turned it on me.

A younger man might have defended himself, defended us, but that day I had no stomach for it. I said nothing further. I climbed the stairs to our bedroom and walked into our bathroom. Now tears overwhelmed me. All around me was evidence of Jack, from the brightly-colored towels to the funny knickknacks on the counter. It was all him. I cupped cold water into my hands to dunk my face. I looked up and saw myself in the mirror, water running off my nose and hair, tears blurring my vision. My face was puffy, my eyes red, my nose running. I brought my hands up to cover my face to bring some relief, some atavistic comfort, with the touch of my own hands. I wanted to tell her that we didn't know when he was infected, no one knew in those years when we had no evidence until it was too late.

But rebellion, not apology, began to well in me. Viv had called my brothers and me perverts, but love and sacrifice can never be perverse. After all the care, all the love we had demonstrated toward our sick and dying brothers, if some people thought us subhuman, let them think so, we weren't ashamed. No longer hiding in shadow, we were standing in the light. The epidemic had furthered what the Stonewall riot had begun—the destruction of our generation had both outed us and revealed our humanity. The price was, and is, far too much and I would not have chosen this, our epidemic. But we had purchased with our lives the right to claim our humanity, and turn shame against those who would shame us.

But I did not go down and tell Viv this. In the end, I left what I had said alone. Saying more would accomplish nothing; it wouldn't change Viv's hostility, or accusation, or anguish. At the last, she allowed a graveside ceremony back in Collinsville. Under the awning at the cemetery, I sat in the front row with his biologic family. But my position was due to the largesse of the Soehlke family, not my obvious prerogative. I sat where I sat because Jack's family wished it so, not because it was Jack's wish.

NEVER AGAIN (I THOUGHT)

When Jack left us, I made a decision that I would never again have a serious relationship with anyone: HIV-positive or HIV-negative. For me, I could have no second Jack, nor would I be someone else's Jack. To be with someone HIV-negative was inconceivable. Whether or not I myself would need eight months of chemotherapy, one thing seemed certain—the day would come when I'd be in a hospital bed in some living room or hospice. Would someone who loved me refuse to leave the room as they zipped the body bag closed? Would some other grieving man be told it was "against policy" for someone else to ride along in the ambulance to the mortuary?

I had been fortunate to have him as long as I did—he had enriched my life and along the way he had created so many trip-wires of memory:

I will never put clothes in a drying machine without his voice in my ear telling me to clean the lint trap *every* time I use a dryer.

I never load a dishwasher without hearing his astonished laughter the day I mistakenly used *regular* dish soap and flooded the kitchen with bubbles.

Each Christmas I remember the gifts unexpectedly presented to me by his family in Collinsville, but which had actually all come from him.

My life is immeasurably richer for the memory of Jack quietly handing me a can of soda when I returned from closing the eyes of another one of our brothers. I had known someone who'd stare across a pillow and tell me of the beauty of a soul struggling with my work. And that I was loved. But our relationship had used every ounce of me—I couldn't do it again. I had loved him and the price had been tremendous. I could not be there for someone else's end; I would not allow someone to be tethered to mine.

THE SEARCH FOR THE MARRIAGE RING

After the 1994 Northridge earthquake, when graffiti began to appear within the walls of the condominium complex, I bought a two-bedroom house tucked inside the Hollywood Hills. In spite of a multitude of neighbors nearby, I looked out the glass wall of my living room and saw only forest. My upstairs had a second bedroom just off the kitchen and it was in this room one day, while watching TV, I took Jack's ring off my finger. (It's a nervous habit of mine that I take a ring off my finger and absent-mindedly play with it). It slipped out of my hand and fell; I bent to pick it up and, to my surprise, it wasn't on the floor. Looking underneath the bed, I found it wasn't there. Not on the bedspread, not in the sheets. My fears escalated as my search widened. Had it rolled into the adjacent guest bathroom? Had it bounced into the sink or bathtub? No. Was it on the windowsill? No. Where could it possibly be? My search was to be repeated in its entirety over the ensuing weeks, and even months. It was not possible, but the ring was lost. Jack's ring, the ring I had promised to wear in his memory, was gone.

In the ensuing months I not only searched for the ring but went to extremes I would not have imagined. One night in a gay bar I bumped into a semi-famous medium. I am firm in my beliefs: I do not believe in hocus-pocus. Nor mediums. Nor, in spite of whatever phenomenon may have happened with my patient with a near-death experience, communication from beyond the grave. But perhaps it was possible, I suddenly imagined, that by some miracle he could divine the location of my, of our, beloved ring. I found myself telling this medium the story of Jack and me, the lost ring and my promise. The answer from the Great Beyond was less than helpful—the medium reported that he didn't work for individual clients anymore. I felt my cheeks redden. I had embarrassed myself for nothing.

Years later, in 1999, I was in the process of moving back to San Francisco when, as the moving truck was full and I made my last walk-through of the house, lightning struck. There, in the center of my one-car garage, was the gold ring, diamond sparkling, unobscured by any debris or rubbish. It was unharmed, undamaged—the same ring I had placed on Jack's finger so many years ago in Venice. One might imagine that I then took that ring and that it never leaves my finger today. But the truth is, while I always know where it is, I only wear it from time to time. For the ring, like all these memories of Jack, my medical training in Seattle and San Francisco, my practice with Lawrence Medical Group, and the 50 patients and friends I walked with to the edge—all these memories have a place in my heart that will never be lost. I have AIDS, which is really just a reminder I carry closely the mortality we all share. A reminder to enjoy every minute and press those around me to do the same. To live in a spirit of gratitude. To make every moment as happy as possible. And to make every moment count. I don't wear Jack's ring every day, just as I don't ponder these memories every day, nor do I reach my goals for everyday happiness. But I have an aim, an ambition, to always live seeing the beauty in the world and in the people I love. To lend my ear and my experiences to those who might desire them, and to be forgiving and gentle with those around me, and myself. And face ahead, not behind.

ANDREW M. FAULK, M.D.

NO WAY TO PARTY

Having left my practice and therefore having the free time, I went to the 1993 White Party (a huge dance event) held every Easter in Palm Springs. There is a perplexing phenomenon, occurring in both heterosexual and homosexual circles, in which a person appears more attractive when they are with someone rather than alone. Of course with this awareness comes the conundrum that one is available when one is without the date that provides the added allure. After Jack's death, I traveled to Palm Springs in the hope that my availability would nevertheless trump my solitude.

Lawrence Medical Group was well known for being an AIDS practice; we advertised ourselves as such in the gay newspaper and LMG regularly purchased entire tables at charity functions. There is a patient's shame with nearly every disease and with AIDS it was worse. With fears and prejudices revolving around HIV everywhere at the time, chance encounters with patients required finesse—for the doctor's oath of doctor-patient confidentiality was always in effect. It was not acceptable for me to greet someone outside the office—for anonymity would be lost if someone were identified as an HIV patient. I found it was never best to acknowledge a patient first but rather wait for the person to greet me and if the individual didn't respond, then I wouldn't say "hello." So it was with these parameters in mind that I attended that year's White Party.

I recognized three patients, separately, among the 3,000 or so attendees that weekend in Palm Springs, or rather three partners of deceased patients. As proper protocol dictated, I studiously awaited signs of recognition from each of them. As each noticed me, it was with a little surprise and some sadness that I detected reservation. The care that their partners had received from me and LMG had been good and I had developed positive relationships with all three, but I found in these survivors a common reluctance to associate with me. I could see it in their eyes: it wasn't that they were concerned they would be taken as AIDS patients, rather it was that my presence reminded them of the difficult and painful episodes they had experienced with their loved ones. I had held their hands in a hellish period of their lives. I had been more than their doctor; I had been their supporter, advocate, champion, and I had been their friend. But I had been these things during one of the worst periods of their lives.

In the end they greeted me but were visibly uncomfortable. They were grateful to me but my presence reminded them of the black period in their lives. And they didn't want to be reminded. They didn't want to be taken back to those dark, brutal times of ER visits at 3:00 a.m., hospital nurses attempting IV lines on worn-out veins, battles with families and insurance companies to keep their loved one comfortable and themselves sane. All in order to ultimately wake up one day exhausted and alone. I understood how the pain of these times made them resistant to being around me. Perhaps there was a part of me that also dreaded their presence.

Our memories were too fresh. Our hearts too bruised.

DARREN AND ANOTHER GOODBYE PARTY

After Jack's death I lived in a haze of loss and anxiety which only increased as it was superseded by the far more formidable fog of HIV encephalopathy. If I had had any doubts about giving up my career, they were laid to rest then. I had free time, but it weighed heavily on me as my own demise seemed close at hand. Without the advent of the "cocktail," there was little to be done other than taking what medications we had at the time and keeping my doctor appointments: the life of a "civilian." But, thankfully, I lived my life as if I had nothing physically wrong—even when a symptom or two would argue against this denial. I was never married to my illness.

Meanwhile life had changed for me. I no longer worked 12 to 16 hours a day. I had enough money—but what use did I have for a savings account?

I bought a set of dining room chairs by my favorite designer Charles Rennie Mackintosh. An Italian company used his original specifications to make reproductions that were beautiful in their design and simplicity. In West Hollywood there is a large complex that houses leading interior design stores and it was in one of several box-like buildings, the "Blue Building," that I found Darren Clark manning the store which sold my chairs. He was in his mid-20s, slender and with a disarming smile and self-effacing demeanor—with just the occasional camp to let you know which team he played on. He moved with the ease and casual grace consistent with his generation, a generation which seemed to have had much less difficulty coming out. I, on the other hand, was of the generation that came of age when Darren's type of openness would have been dangerous to career, social standing and living situation—if not physical safety.

For we were largely either mistrusted or despised or both and the surrounding society offered no sympathy or protection. If we were lucky, we saw the more or less outrageous public personalities of people like Charles Nelson Reilly, Paul Lynde and, perhaps, Quentin Crisp, although never Harry Hay. But the world in which Darren Clark came of age seemed largely free of the hysteria and harsh judgments of the old. One of the things I love about California is the comfortable and matter-of-fact attitude with which society accepted us—sometimes grudgingly, but accepting all the same. For the Golden State was part of the changing national *zeitgeist* and it was surprising and refreshing, albeit disconcerting in its novelty, to swim in a sea rapidly changing in temperature and current.

After studying the different Mackintosh chairs available, I returned a third time to Darren's showroom. He invited me to his back office where we had a coke as he filled out the required forms and I wrote a check. During the three months it took to have the chairs manufactured, he changed from a healthy-looking man, although thin, to one emaciated and gray. Upon hearing that I was an AIDS doctor, he questioned me regarding the quality of care his own physician was providing. I assured him that his doctor was more than capable. The disease was so little understood, the field so new, that when questioned about the quality of other doctors, I only expressed doubts when someone limited their care to Chinese herbs, acupuncture, chiropractic or there was enough information to label the provider a quack. When my chairs were eventually delivered, Darren invited me back to his office for a celebratory drink.

His disease had progressed rapidly. His face now showed the typical seborrheic dermatitis, the all-too-common bi-temporal wasting and the bronze skin of adrenal failure. Jack's death had left me stunned with little emotion and little to say and I was not tempted to offer any false hope—Darren knew his future. Fortunately for my own nerves, he spoke easily, at first about a memory of camping with his late father and then about his own approaching death. He had decided to have a Goodbye Party; he had several credit cards with a significant amount of available credit and had already rented a "presidential" suite at a hotel in West Hollywood. He was inviting his friends to the farewell. Although these farewells ended with what appeared to be the person drifting off "to sleep," I couldn't help but see these grim get-togethers as barely-hidden violence.

I am well-educated in the last stages of this illness. While, obviously, not philosophically opposed to doctor-assisted euthanasia, for myself I find preparation and execution of it too distressing to imagine. I stress, as any good clinician will, that it's not to be aided if the person is experiencing depression or dementia. In spite of this I hope that I myself will find the courage for suicide or, rather, physician-assisted suicide, should my disease progress along certain paths. At the top of my list is PML—progressive multifocal leukoencephalopathy. But I make no promises—to myself or others—about the sunset of my life. My medical power of attorney is instructed to approve the continuation of care as long as I am capable of enjoying existence. But when it comes to suicide, I don't make concrete commitments. In the end I may be hysterical, although I hope not. Rather, I trust I will confront the final moments of life with serenity and dignity. And I hope that should I develop one of the diseases on my short list, I will have the foresight and fortitude to take my life by my own hand. But the decision and preparation for the endeavor I find emotionally overwhelming and I suspect I will allow inertia to choose my end.

I've experienced several kinds of Goodbye Parties—each tremendously different from the others and having its own individual anxiety and sorrow. This one seemed to lack the underlying sad desperation of the others I'd been to. The hotel suite Darren chose was very large with a bedroom, sitting room and huge bathroom. Darren loved flowers and there were so many bouquets and "falls" that one might have thought the death had already occurred. Ironically, there was no marijuana smoking as it was a non-smoking room in a non-smoking hotel. Although it was a day for breaking the rules, the gravity of the event made the participants oddly careful at first. Later, they opened the windows and relaxed the rules and their tensions as they smoked both tobacco and marijuana. We obtained some visual relief from the extraordinarily handsome bartenders who were not, at least at first, aware of the true nature of the event. Darren had hired a group of five guys to sing who were wonderfully upbeat and campy. Their songs dealt, as one might think, with the difficulty of our orientation. Although they were the most cheerful people in the room, they had to have known the purpose of the event.

I went to the hotel alone and didn't spend more than 10 minutes with Darren. I used the excuse that my M.D. license would be in jeopardy should I stay while he took the medication. I don't know whether Darren believed me; but he certainly went along with the premise. He had already taken something and his eyes were just a little glazed. On each side of him sat two friends he had chosen to be with him when he took the final dose. It seemed almost out of place, but I told Darren, as I had stressed with my own patients who had chosen this route, that should he have a change of mind at any point, 911 could be dialed and medical personnel could interrupt the effect of the medications. (Obviously I didn't mention the nasogastric stomach pumping.) "Don't worry about it, Dr. Faulk, I'm okay with this," he understated. He had never called me "Dr. Faulk" before.

Although Darren was not my patient, I felt the impact of this Goodbye Party through and through. At the others, being the person's doctor had inexplicably left me more detached. I cried alone in the hotel bathroom that afternoon, with my forehead pressed against the cold, ceramic wall. Crying seems to focus and distill free-floating sorrow as nothing else can, perhaps that's why we often feel better after the tears have come. When I left the hotel suite that afternoon, however, the "party" had left me shaken to my core.

MICHAEL TAYLOR AND JOHN SWENSON

When I was still in practice, Jack and I were friends with the couple John Swenson, my patient, and his partner Michael Taylor. Jack and I had been invited to their house for dinner during the Christmas season of 1990 and it is another gathering in which I share the memory with only one other person—Michael. John and he had been wonderfully supportive with delivered meals and drop-in visits when Jack was dying, but within five months of Jack's passing, John, too, was dead. His mother had been one of those parents who continued a relationship with their fallen son's partner and the two of them threw a memorial gathering that first Christmas after he passed away. I was invited but mostly I stood alone, speaking a little with only those few who knew me and felt comfortable around my silence. In any case, Michael and I lost contact after that.

Eight years later in 1999, when I moved back to San Francisco with then-partner Lance, I stumbled upon a letter from Michael dated sometime during the period 1991 through 1993 when the years after Jack's death were the most foggy. The letter, sadly, had never been opened. I'm ashamed to say that Michael's letter was mostly about my inaccessibility. He was angry—we had been friends, he thought, and I had become unreachable.

Obviously, a great deal of patient care depends upon availability. While I was in practice I was, of course, almost constantly available. However the confluence of my own illness, grief at Jack's passing, and the loss of my medical career was an emotional cataclysm to which I reacted by withdrawing from much of the world. Except for the easily discernible bills, I would go weeks without opening mail. A letter could mean news of another death or it could be a request, something which I'd need to act upon. I told myself that I would tackle the mail in a few days, when I was feeling stronger emotionally. I couldn't stand the contact, the shared memories. I was no different than the partners of my patients at Palm Springs' White Parties who couldn't stand the memories I evoked.

Whether it be ground mail, e-mail or phone, with all the energy of an obsessive-compulsive disorder I avoided communication. Similar to PTSD in its effect, this fear, no matter how irrational, follows me to this day. No matter the inconvenience and potential for catastrophe, I prefer sending letters and postcards instead of engaging in phone calls and e-mail because this one-way communication seemingly protects me from the possibility of bad news.

ANDREW M. FAULK, M.D.

JOHN EMBRY—
FESTIVAL OF CAMP AND BEDROCK OF SUPPORT

John Embry was a loud, funny, over-the-top patient who was always a festival of camp and a source of heart-felt assistance to the men he accompanied into my office. His caring was as tangible as his presence. He would often stand with a hand on each hip in the fashion of a wronged drag queen. He had come from Texas, but his chivalry and Texan dialect were the only things left, apparently, of the prudery and convention which surely had been his upbringing. His cultured choice of words made him extraordinarily entertaining and immediately identified him as a son of the South—although in his case more of a disorderly step-child than a bonafide offspring. He punned incessantly, almost always in the direction of the sordid and lascivious and had that *joie de vivre* which comes from knowing one's *vivre* may disappear any day. I must have met him the first week I worked at LMG and, when I initially walked into that exam room in Los Angeles, he was laughing loudly while the assistant took his vitals. When we were alone, he gleefully asked me if I had been "warned" about him by the other docs. I had not been forewarned, but his statement had the quality of a challenge I was not going to let slide. "No, but what would they have said, John?"

"That I'm a loud queer, that I have a lot of friends and that my jewelry is spectacular!"

He hoped to dumbfound me. During the first few months of my practice at LMG, I usually went to work wearing a tie which, together with my thin frame, thick head of hair and glasses, gave me a somewhat bookish, naïve appearance which was misleading.

Intrigued but noncommittal I said, "Oh, is that right?"

He was grinning from ear to ear. "You want to see them, Doc?"

"Of course," I responded.

At that point he unzipped his jeans, took down his shorts, and showed me what he was obviously proud of—and indeed should have been. Along the midline of the underside of his penis was a neat row of eight to ten small, short rods all neatly arranged equidistant apart (a "frenum ladder").

I was the new doctor in the office and John was testing my squeamish meter. But the gleam of the tiny balls on each side of every stud, so neat and orderly, had me. Whatever he may have anticipated I was going to say, I could tell he was disappointed with my response. "How do you get through security at the airport, John?"

Without missing a beat, he answered, "I ask them if I can take my pants off."

"And do they ask you to take your pants off?"

"Nope, Doc, unfortunately they never do."

My unruffled demeanor simultaneously dissatisfied him and provoked his interest. At the time piercings and tattoos appealed more to the "wild child" in me than my appearance may have suggested, but I didn't want to be identified outside of the "geek" classification I had come to encourage. I preferred to fly underneath the radar. I still do.

But John had attributes far more beguiling than his penile accoutrements: he didn't judge anyone who didn't judge him and he was a rock of support to many of our patients. Although I may not have been outwardly moved by his unconventional ornamentation, he won my quiet admiration by occasionally attending his friend's medical appointments with them—and sometimes even attending office visits with people he barely knew. He provided a remarkable comedic presence at their various tests and hospitalizations. To many, some as equally perforated as himself, he gave physical and emotional support to which they had little access. To those who were newly facing the sobering kitchen blender of medical jargon and laboratory metrics, his presence and ribald jokes gave enormous comfort and battled crushing anxiety. He was a rock for these men and I soon understood that he was well up to the task of walking my guys into the emotional abyss of their HIV infection and, indeed, off

ANDREW M. FAULK, M.D.

the edge of the world. In many, many cases, I knew if John were in the room I could move on to those who were without any support.

Our friendship grew and soon I knew him well enough to visit his home. He had lost a significant number of friends—at their bedsides I imagine. In his living room, on break-fronts and tables, shelves and windowsills, one could see photo after photo of smiling men who received his remarkable attention before dying. These photos included three of his deceased partners.

As his jewelry indicated he was more than a little eccentric, managing a stockbroker business from his kitchen. Monitoring the results of the experimental HIV treatments of which he was aware, he would invest for himself and his friends in those pharmaceutical companies producing what appeared to be the anti-HIV candidates most likely to succeed.

In this winter of loss and sorrow which petrified the hearts of so many, mine to a varying degree among them, John's heart beat constant and strong. He didn't just look after patients. He was one of the few patients who inquired after me personally. I saw him on and off through my years at LMG and our mutual affection and presence in the holocaust raging around us kept us connected. As it happened, he was never a guest at our house when Jack was alive, but he made charming and provocative appearances during the few get-togethers I had at the condo after Jack passed away.

THE LAST WISH OF DAVID ST. GEORGE

Leaving the practice left me a haunted man. I was at a loss—I had surrendered my career, but I wasn't dead and there was still fight left in me. I could still contribute, perhaps not as a physician, but in some other meaningful way. John, well-known for his ability to network, referred me to David St. George, a man living in Albuquerque who was nearing the end of his life. David lived alone and had no one to provide him care or companionship. I knew I wasn't in a position to provide medical care, but I knew I could provide the presence of someone with medical training.

David flew out to Los Angeles to see me and we immediately hit it off. He had been an attorney and was a short, slight figure, with a reserved, quiet manner; he was the exact antithesis of boisterous John Embry. It seemed he had no friends except casual acquaintances and, of course, John.

David was thankful and, more than anything, joyous about my coming to stay with him for a while. He had the same illness as I: AIDS encephalopathy—disorder of the brain caused by HIV and often ending in an Alzheimer's-like picture. It wasn't anything new for me to spend time with someone who had my diagnosis and be confronted with symptoms which I might very well develop. I knew these possibilities well. There was nothing new to fear.

His house in Albuquerque was spacious and comfortable and when I arrived, I saw his calendar marked "Andrew arrives TODAY!" Once moved in, the time slipped away with tourist visits to Native American villages and nearby Santa Fe. I hadn't been there long when David told to me his one last wish: he wanted to see Amsterdam. He was afraid his health wouldn't permit a trip to Europe but this seemed like exactly the function for which I was there. There were to be complications—upon returning from a quick trip to L.A. for my passport, I found his encephalopathy had worsened and he was able to walk only with great difficulty. Together we saw his primary M.D. and discussed it there in the office and, as his mentation was nearly unaffected, we decided to go ahead with his wish.

Soon we were packing and on our way, but it was an inauspicious beginning. The trans-Atlantic flight was incredibly difficult because I hadn't made arrangements for us to sit near the toilets. With other passengers staring in disbelief and sympathy, I physically carried David, in a "dead man" carry, back and forth to the restroom. It was an experience I hope never to repeat. Nothing could have been sweeter, however, after the horrendous plane trip than the excitement of Amsterdam. This was David's "last hurrah" and so the hotel was first-rate, the restaurants terrific and we soon had tickets to see a famous play then being performed there.

But we hadn't been there long when he developed fevers and a dry cough. I knew the likely diagnosis and quickly took him to a hospital. His chest X-ray showed the typical blanket of snow and he was immediately admitted with the diagnosis of *Pneumocystis* pneumonia. Although I looked over the shoulders of the doctors providing his care, I had little to add or question. Dutch medicine was state-of-the-art and Dutch doctors more than competent. With David hospitalized I soon fell into a pattern in which I would leave the hotel mid-morning and spend the rest of the day with him in the hospital—I saw very little of the Netherlands besides hospital corridors.

Toward the end of his hospitalization, David's sister flew out from Chicago. She was nearly our age, easy going and fun to be around and she brought a lightness into the hospital room and into the trip. Her presence allowed me to see some of the city, although David was on my mind even when I was sightseeing and she was with him. She couldn't have shown me more appreciation while we were together there in Amsterdam. After about two weeks of treatment, his pneumonia cleared but his mental status remained clouded and he stayed hospitalized another two weeks. The three of us returned to New Mexico where his sister decided to move in with him. It was while I was unpacking him I came upon a bombshell—there at the bottom of one of his suitcases I found to my perfect consternation a plastic bag filled with cocaine! He had packed on his own before the trip and I hadn't seen it. Customs must have judged his condition too grave for us to be worthy of a thorough search for we had passed inspection in two countries. Here I was, taking charge of our entry papers and luggage when all the while we were carrying with us cocaine and a prison sentence!

With David's sister assuming his care, I returned to L.A. In about 10 days I received a strange call from a confused David asking for my forgiveness—for what did I need to forgive? He was too muddled to say, but it was related to his will. I "forgave" him quickly and our phone conversation ended soon after. I didn't hear anything more from him or his sister so I assumed HIV had taken its course.

A month later I ran into John who let me know David had died within a week of his phone call to me. He had slipped into a coma and drifted away. What surprised me was John's report that, in that last week, I had been removed from his will which had originally bequeathed me $200,000. I hadn't known I was in his testament—nor had I expected to be. Evidently David's sister had taken advantage of his confusion to persuade him to change his will at the last moment and leave everything to her. John's friend, John Li, had also been cut out of the will, but had gone to court, without any success, and discovered the various amounts David's friends were to have received. As I'd extrapolated my T-cell numbers and surmised I'd be dead in a year or two, what did money matter? But I was nonetheless touched that he had thought of me.

The story of wills being changed at the last moment was commonplace. Several of my friends and patients feared their relatives would push them to change their wills when they were incapacitated. It was not an unjustified fear; I was to hear this scenario repeated again and again.

I went on to provide companionship and care for two other men with AIDS living in Los Angeles—Thomas Harrington and Gabriel Hernandez. As before with David St. George I moved in with them and, for these men with neither relatives nor close friends, I provided supervision in taking their medications, a helping hand to wash and clean and a calming presence to talk them down when the terrors of the night became too great. Both died within three weeks of my beginning to live with them.

After these times, my emotions were burnt and it was clear to me, I had done what I could do. I could no longer serve in any way.

DANIEL JAMES

John Embry was more than a friend—through all the fog of grief, I remember he and Linda Gromko attending Jack's funeral. Six months after Jack's death, when I was still living in a twilight of sorrow and near-total isolation, I called him and asked him to go to a bar with me. On the phone I said, "Listen, John, I need to be with people tonight. Could we meet at a bar or something? We don't have to talk about Jack or anybody else that's gone. Just hang out." Really, any environment would have been acceptable, but if we happened to drift into the storm, a guy crying in a gay bar wasn't the spectacle it might have been elsewhere.

After Jack was gone and I was no longer in practice, I found myself standing in bars far too much. The hours wasted, I'm afraid, were substantial and on my deathbed, should I complain about lack of time, I need to remind myself that I wasted precious time in bars during these years. Just the presence of gay guys around me, however, provided a mental respite and, of course, a feeling of physical safety.

That night John and I chatted about the superficial things people talk about in bars. Neither of us wanted to discuss a mutual friend's death that had occurred the preceding week. But after some time had passed with no words being exchanged between us, he walked over to the bar, found a writing pad, wrote something down and returned to the emotional safety the bar wall provided. He handed me a slip of paper with the name "Daniel James" and a telephone number. "Call him up" John said, "Dating isn't marriage." I took the piece of paper.

Although Daniel was known as "Bink" to his friends, I could never attach that name to him. He was shorter and younger than I, red-haired and small-boned. His smile confirmed his introversion which nonetheless had enough warmth to make one feel they were noticed and accepted. He had a hearing impairment and wore a hearing aid in his left ear and, if one listened closely, they could hear the slight mispronunciation of those consonants difficult for the hearing-impaired to master. Nevertheless in a quiet environment he could hear much, if not most, conversation but he also relied on lip reading and, simplified for me, sign language. In spite of this obstacle we managed together quite well and to my quiet satisfaction he once remarked that none of his previous boyfriends had engaged him in conversation as much as I did. He was a handsome man but in the competitive physicality of late 20th century Los Angeles my insecurities made me worry that my looks were inferior to his. His matter-of-fact acceptance of our difficulty in communication, however, made me believe I was allowed a pass in this respect.

Perhaps because of his hearing impediment he was insightful and quick to identify people's qualities. In general he had a way of emphasizing the good and minimizing the bad that was often infuriating. The fact that he happened to be red-haired, as I am, aggravated my own internal homophobic prejudice that most gay couples appear to be nearly identical. But never mind. Daniel had had a problematic childhood, I knew, but he didn't speak of his family. To this day I know of no details of his childhood or youth or, for that matter, any relatives. It was as if he had no history before we met. Such breaks with the past were not unusual in gay circles and not particularly outlandish.

When I was in high school, my Evangelical Lutheran church routinely sponsored a summer camp for disabled children in British Columbia. It was there that I learned some simple sign language and how to spell. Years later my training was sufficient for uncomplicated conversation and therefore I saw all of LMG's deaf patients. For those many situations in which my vocabulary was inadequate, I was still effective because, after all, one can spell *anything*. But Daniel preferred us not to use sign language in public; he didn't like the visible exhibition of his impairment. So in public he lip-read when he could, and nodded assent when he couldn't. There are hard of hearing people who develop a method of navigating in the world which reinforces a distinctive and secretly disparaging exclusivity, but that was not his way and he was happy to draw others in.

He used to proudly repeat "I have no regrets" as his personal mantra. As he frequently and adamantly stated this axiom, I pondered its meaning—both in my own life and in Dan's. Did he consider all mistakes to be intolerable personality flaws or unforgivable judgment blunders? Or perhaps the opposite was occurring—maybe he narcissistically saw all negative events as originating outside himself. Contrary to Shakespeare, did he absolve himself by concluding that the faults in our lives do, in fact, lie in our stars? In retrospect, I believe this was a choice he had made in which he refused to punish himself for anything in his past. He saw no benefit in looking back; perhaps he reasoned that there was enough grief in the present. In my life, however, I've done much learning and growing up through mistakes and the regret they engender. And past regret has done much to side-step future blunders. When Frank or I consider pushing the "send" button on some text late in the evening, we ask ourselves whether we will regret what we've said in the morning; we specifically use the word "regret" in our analysis. Recognition of past mistakes, for me, is a productive tool in building self-awareness and avoiding *creating* wrongs in the future. I think Dan saw regret only as crippling sorrow instead of a productive mechanism for avoiding future mistakes. Shortly after moving to San Francisco, Lance accidentally threw my only suit in the washing machine and it came out perfectly fitted for a hobbit. Instead of apologizing for this rather minor flaw in attention, he was adamant that he was *not* going to feel bad or apologize for the misstep! I suspect some of the same narcissistic dynamic was in play there as with Daniel. Beyond the irritating message telling me that his feelings were more important than mine, my intuition told me that any future suit I might have would live in constant jeopardy. For he saw no benefit in feeling remorse for past errors—they were only unhelpful self-abuse.

In spite of my resistance to getting close to anyone, I remembered John's aphorism about dating not being marriage and enjoyed Daniel as we began spending more time together. But knowing his HIV status, I admit I kept a certain distance. And over time I began to notice an unattractive inclination that some of my brothers, or anyone, without resources occasionally display—the vigorous and often loud expectation of the best in accommodations as well as finding fault with superlative service. Besides this predilection, Daniel had a manipulative mind-set that didn't shirk from using people and situations to achieve his goals. He principally employed fact-bending and small deceptions, but lies are lies and by paying attention I learned more than he intended: if he'd use a friend, I determined, he'd use me. In hearing matters of dishonor, an attentive listener should only presume he is an exception at his own peril.

The experience of my years taught me that such a character failing could not be adjusted with a simple heart-to-heart conversation. Or many such discussions. Had I allowed myself to become more deeply involved, there would have been non-HIV problems partnering with Daniel. When he developed subtle changes of abdominal lipodystrophy and bitemporal wasting, I ended the relationship definitively. Our break-up was inevitable, but the timing was excruciating.

Daniel moved to San Francisco and I didn't—at least not at that time. Making myself unavailable for bad news by mail or telephone, I didn't keep in touch with him, but a mutual friend later told me that Dan had died in the spring of 1995. He spent the last year of his life as an impoverished recluse living in a friend's garage. He didn't live to see his 37th birthday.

THE DEATH OF NORMAN NASH

About the time I was breaking up with Daniel I found myself back in touch with New Jersey friend Norman Nash who had also lost his partner of a decade in the late '80s. In the spring of 1993 we went to the third National March on Washington together and there, unfortunately, we had a falling-out. He disapproved of a couple of new acquaintances I had made and destroyed their business cards. He had become too protective of me, smothering me in the process, and I ended up withdrawing from him. We hadn't had an argument, I simply drifted away. This is a regret in my life because it robbed me of that last bit of time I could have enjoyed with him. It was a sad miscalculation in my life because it was that September that Norman called. His T-cells had been dropping, he said, and he'd begun to lose weight. He called to say he was dying. My first words were, "No you're not." I tried to quiet him; I told him he was overreacting. While my training and experience may have agreed with him, I simply didn't want to face his death. Another person close to me couldn't die. I spoke to make myself feel better, not Norman. It was a common phenomenon: many people who discourage the ill from frankly discussing their disease have similar motives. They want to ease their own pain. Here I was no different.

"No," he replied, "I'm having constant diarrhea." I can no longer remember my words, I must have told him to have it evaluated. A few weeks later, I got a call from George Jones, his best friend, telling me that Norman was hospitalized in a community hospital near his home in Elizabeth, New Jersey. He was not thought to survive long. I flew to New York.

Norman was in a near-coma state, but his grimaces, moans

and spikes in heart rate and blood pressure let us know he was suffering. Perianal herpes, which he had, is well known to cause bone-wrenching pain. There was no way I was going to let my buddy experience this degree of agony, especially when we have good tools for treatment. I went to the nurses' station and, ethical or not, amongst the diligent hyperactivity of the nurses and doctors, I found Norman's chart and read his medication orders. He was limited to Tylenol. No doubt out of concern that stronger pain control might suppress his blood pressure and respiration to the point his life would be threatened, his doctor was under-treating his pain. It's a common unfortunate misjudgment of a doctor not taking a patient's probable life-span into account when treating pain. I telephoned his Attending physician and gave her my best "come-let-us-reason-together" tone. Annoyed that her care was being questioned, she nevertheless agreed to take several of my suggestions under advisement—but after this discussion Norman's pain medications didn't change. Seeing him in such needless agony hour after hour, I first requested that his private doctor be called by the nursing staff and then, in succession, his nurse and then the charge nurse responsible for the unit he was on. Time passed without intervention. His Attending didn't come to examine him and I asked the staff to once again call her. Perhaps they called, but at this point the entire staff was annoyed with me. I didn't care. Who was I, they asked, a member of the family? "No, not exactly, but a good friend who was a physician," I replied. It was about 3:00 p.m. when a pain order came in from his doctor. We waited while the hospital pharmacy filled the prescription and the nurse piggy-backed the clear fluid into his IV. A morphine drip usually signifies "comfort care"—care to treat nothing more than pain. Norman had just turned 47 and it's difficult for any doctor to place someone on comfort care at such a relatively young age. But it was a time when many, many young men, men younger than Norman, were being placed on comfort care.

Once the morphine drip had begun, a great calm descended on Norman: his thrashing and moaning ended. After having treated strangers for years, I was able to give Norman, this close friend, the benefit of my years of training and experience—and help resolve some of his pain.

It was about 3:30 p.m. I looked out of Norman's window down at the hospital's entrance. It was mid-October; it hadn't snowed yet but it was bitterly cold just the same. Norman was in a twilight state of near consciousness, principally because of the morphine for which I'd fought so hard. His eyes were closed. Suddenly from the hospital bed, he began to speak slowly, but clearly, "The Lord is my Shepherd, I shall not want. He makes me lie down in green pastures. He leads me beside still waters. He restores my soul. He leads me in paths of righteousness for His name's sake…" Startled, George and I looked at him, looked at each other, and then looked back at Norman. Although Jewish, he had never been a religious man. I knew the 23rd Psalm from years of church and Bible camp, and he recited it in its entirety. We were stunned. Over the years, he generously had paid for his nieces to attend Jewish camp in the summers, but that would have had nothing to do with his recitation of the Psalm in English. We weren't prepared for this.

By then the disease had taken a heavy toll on his body. He looked gaunt and frail, with eyes shrunk into their orbits and arms so thin they appeared as if merely shaking his hand might break bones. In this disease, one might expect that with the tremendous transformation of bodies, voices might similarly be affected. A surprising phenomenon, however, was how little damage the voices of those with AIDS underwent, staying as deep and vibrant as before their illness. A person's physical presence may change beyond recognition, it seems, but their voice remains unaltered. Norman's recitation had been in his usual deep voice that we knew so well.

I looked at Norman in that hospital bed; finally, with pain medication, he was soon quietly sleeping. Suddenly, it seemed, it was 6:00 p.m. and two security guards appeared at the door of Norman's room. They each had questions and *guns*. Was I a relative or a friend? I turned toward Norman's friend George who gave me a surprised look. "No," I said, "I'm a close personal friend who happens to be an AIDS physician." One of the security officers placed a hand on his hip, and with a dark, cold look in his eyes said, "Visiting hours are over and you're not a relative. It's time for you to leave the hospital." He had said "hospital" and not "room." Evidently my thoughts on Norman's care hadn't been entirely appreciated. I walked between the two security guards to the elevator, through the lobby and out the front door. I guess they thought the presence of firearms was necessary to give me sufficient incentive to leave.

I was angry in my impotence, however. It was obvious to me

ANDREW M. FAULK, M.D.

Norman wasn't receiving optimum care, especially when it came to pain management. He'd fallen victim to inadequate pain control: pain isn't sufficiently treated for fear the treatment might result in either narcotic addiction—irrelevant in these situations—or the death of the patient due to respiratory and/or cardiac arrest. The first is a destructive overlap of medical ignorance and the dictatorial politics of Puritanical conceit and the second is lack of a broad overview of the patient's pain in light of his or her probable lifespan. In any case, I was with Norman two days that last week of his life, and I'd been successful in easing his pain. Norman died the day after my birthday.

THE COCKTAIL AND ME

I lived to see the advent of the miracle-working antiretroviral "cocktail" (two or more medications—three in my case) which became the norm by 1996. This scientific achievement marked an incredible turning point for those with HIV. For me particularly, because of its effect on my cognition and presumptive lifespan. Before combination antiretroviral therapy, my T-cells (CD4 cells)[1] had been fluctuating in the fairly healthy 350 to 700 range, and since the new medications began there has been no change in my counts. Before, in the late 1980s, I had been tracking my T-cells and had extrapolated their decline; by 1991 I was preparing myself to die in 1993 or 1994. But my counts never fell below 350 and, after 1995, highly active antiretroviral therapy (HAART) kept my T-cells in this elevated range which sustains my general health. It is a testament to these new medications that, some thirty years later, I am still alive. Since needing to leave my practice, I've been most pained by my impaired cognition—that is, my thinking and memory. But in 2001 my HIV encephalopathy, with predictably intermittent setbacks, slowly began to improve. This is an unbelievable phenomenon, unheard of in HIV medicine, and almost certainly due to the advancement in medications. Because of the characteristic limitations of the brain, and the aggressive nature of the virus, this is one of the most astonishing facts of my story.

    Parenthetically, I also attribute the pronounced improvement in

1 The T-cell count (CD4 count) is the laboratory test generally accepted as the best indicator of the immediate state of immunologic competence of those with HIV infection. I have used lone numbers for T-cell counts (e.g., "200") when, in actuality, I mean the number of CD4 T-cells per cubic mm. A normal CD4 T-cell count is 500/cubic mm to 1,200/cubic mm.

ANDREW M. FAULK, M.D.

my thinking, in part, to being placed on amphetamine combinations (e.g., Adderall)—this improved reasoning is the only thing I actually feel. By contributing to my cognition, amphetamines have markedly improved my quality of life.

The experience of losing some 50 patients and friends, along with my perpetual vulnerability, has left me with something very close to Post Traumatic Stress Disorder. PTSD is well known to produce, among other things, major depression and social withdrawal. In my medical career my shadowed imagination registered the possibility, the probability, of my becoming, sometime in the unkind future, every patient I examined. These are not trivial fears. But they, and my PTSD, have thankfully decreased over time—I've become better able to remember instead of relive.

In spite of the cocktail, however, I frequently experience painfully unpredictable episodes of diarrhea which may be due to HIV or the medications or a combination of both. And my tremors increasingly look like a type of Parkinson's Disease which, like the diarrhea, may have something to do with HIV or the medications or the two in conjunction. Luckily an atypical speech disorder, which occasionally rendered me near mute, responds well to medications. One cannot predict, however, how these symptoms may have evolved had I not been on the cocktail.

But there are occasions when memory deficits and word searching are frustrating, and it's rare for me to be with anyone who has lived through the epidemic, especially a physician, so when I'm with people there's often a part of me that feels alone and isolated.

The beginning of HAART was a tremendous breakthrough which leaves me with tremendous hope. The anti-viral cocktail, in consistently maintaining my T-cell count above 350, has radically amplified my cognition. But CD4 counts above 200 don't protect one from nerve issues such as peripheral neuropathy and I realize the longer I live the more susceptible I become to my uneven mentation deteriorating into AIDS dementia. For me the effect of the cocktail is that the pool may be far less deep, but I'm still treading water.

Whether living with almost no hope, as before the new anti-HIV cocktail, or much hope, as now, my emotional outlook has remained consistent: I ignore my AIDS diagnosis. I think of it as "ignoring" as opposed to "denying" for I diligently take my medications four times a day and faithfully keep doctor appointments and instructions. For someone less schooled in HIV, an elevated and stable T-cell count would be ample reassurance. In the small hours of the night, though—when life is the most bleak—I struggle with the paradox of knowing too much in a world in which information is usually empowerment. Even while experiencing some HIV symptoms, however, even while taking all these medications throughout the day, I don't live in an awareness that these intrusions are due to an underlying illness. Oddly enough, this doesn't seem to be as difficult as one might imagine: I'm largely successful at emotionally discounting the various symptoms and my medication schedule as routine—merely the "price of doing business." Crucially, I'm not married to my illness.

ANDREW M. FAULK, M.D.

THE RELATIONSHIP WITH LANCE

Lance Newman entered my life by way of an improbable blind date. In those days between 1995 and 1998, I spent an inordinate amount of time in bars attempting to escape the shadows and whispers filling my head. One night in the early spring of 1998, as I was standing alone in a Silverlake bar, I was approached by an exuberant, heavy man with red hair and a beard to match, introducing himself as David. He hit on me and I told him thank you very much, but no, he wasn't my "type." Usually that would be enough to end further discussion but my new acquaintance persisted, "Well then, what's your type?" After pondering the down-side of airing such personal information, I told David those preferences I was comfortable giving and we parted.

Weeks later I was in the same bar when David surfaced. "Listen, I've got a guy for you." Having forgotten our earlier conversation, I couldn't imagine what he was talking about. "You know," he said excitedly, "I found someone who matches your list and whose list matches you! I have his phone number right here!" Yes, a date and I were to be introduced by a perfect stranger who knew almost nothing about either of us.

Lance and I ultimately met in a Los Angeles restaurant and clicked as David and I had not. He was dark, handsome, and my ideal in many ways—a sexy man with intelligence, education and an ease in living in his own skin. Before the advent of the highly active antiretroviral cocktail, Lance had been profoundly ill and, as a matter of fact, continued to suffer painful neuropathy. I was comfortable with him—he understood the struggle with HIV.

For a time, however, I was wracked with worry that I was

putting myself at risk for the exhaustion and heartache of walking another partner off the edge of the world—perhaps trauma I might not survive a second time. Eventually though I made the conscious decision to ignore my fears as they were borne of an immutable history and, instead, resuscitate hope and nurture its survival as a counterweight to these terrors. For I realized that when the range of possibilities are considered honestly both safety and jeopardy are illusion. I reasoned that perhaps I could place confidence in myself to withstand the punishing maelstrom of another partner's long walk off the earth. For whatever strength and resilience I had developed had been forged in that same furnace as my fears, and thus had in them that same durability.

While I had fully lived the emotional pandemonium of the epidemic, I dreamt of a sustained period of calmer, happier times enjoyed with a partner. I didn't want my relationship with Jack, wonderful as it was, to permanently demarcate the parameters of my life; I wanted my time with him to merely color a piece in its spectrum. Whether it was to be an illness of Lance's or an illness of mine, I would make a leap of faith that either would be manageable. And should I be the first to sicken, I would have the experience of someone else pushing my wheelchair, holding a bucket while I retched, cleaning my soiled sheets, and washing my bedpan. It would be a shattering lesson in surrender and humility, but hopefully one I would transcend.

In any case, David had struck gold for me: in a matter of weeks strangers were asking how many years Lance and I had been together. In January of 1999, Lance and I exchanged vows before an attorney and friends, signed domestic partnership papers, and celebrated with the fizz of champagne!

Our relationship grew until Lance and I traveled east to Philadelphia to visit an old girlfriend of his. Above her home office desk was a photograph of Lance when he was at his medical worst; I was horrified to see him in the pale, emaciated state of someone with advanced disease. Previously I thought I had come to a point of accepting an exacerbation in his illness, but this photo created an emotional shock which hijacked my thoughts of any future for us. For me our thriving relationship suddenly withered and in the space of a few hours became untenable. In spite of my concordat with hope, I simply couldn't do this again—I couldn't nurse another partner through his passing. After an extremely strained month, however, the beauty of his loving support and companionship calmed my emotions. I never told Lance of this crisis, how could I? And when our relationship eventually did end, fear of an impending holocaust of illness and grief didn't play a part. Lance and I had had an extraordinary relationship, but no break-up goes well and ours was no exception. On St. Patrick's Day, 2004, Lance moved the last of his things out of our apartment. In spite of the wisdom in separating, I was seriously bruised.

But that was years later. Early in our relationship, San Francisco beckoned. Besides perfect weather (without the constant, oppressive sun, heat and traffic of L.A.), at the turn of the last century it was one of the most gay-friendly cities in America. In San Francisco one was presumed to be gay just as often as not. By late 1999 Lance and I were settling down in its famous gay neighborhood, the Castro. I began to sculpt, and then work in mixed media, while Lance pursued his astrology and, happily for me, cooking. We bought a house on the Russian River in Guerneville. I was happier than I'd been in years.

LOUIS AND THE WORK-WORLD BATTLE

It was about the time when I had just moved back to San Francisco from L.A. when I heard from Louis Bryan whom I knew from my days as an intern. Louis, who had lost his lover Allen more than a decade earlier, had planned a dinner for me and Lance. Louis was a busy man, with many friends and commitments, so our get-together had been scheduled weeks in advance. Yet when Lance and I arrived for dinner, we found him in a state of anguished panic. He had forgotten our dinner entirely, and was despondent; he had just returned from the office where he worked and had walked out without notifying his team, or even turning his computer off—a "dot-com sin." Louis, who as a tech writer translated computerese into English, had been experiencing more and more difficulty performing his work until that very day when he had been overwhelmed by its complexity and his own failing skills. Beside himself with confusion and despair, Louis was bewildered as to how he could continue such intellectually-demanding work. He was pacing and rubbing his breastbone compulsively and one could easily hear his Texas dialect.

It was clear to Lance and me that, like so many other friends, patients, and, indeed, both of ourselves, his working days were over. To lose such an enormous battle in our struggle against the virus was a crushing, but necessary, realization. Often one's friends played a part in acceptance—Dr. Feraru had done as much for me. I sat Louis down and asked him to concentrate on what I was about to say: "Louis," I said, "this is it for you. All of us reach a point where we can no longer work, and attempting to prolong our occupation only makes the situation worse." Louis' mouth gaped in stunned disbelief. "Think, Louis, how overwhelmed you are now. Stress exacerbates

ANDREW M. FAULK, M.D.

HIV. Think of the pressure you'd avoid if you faced the truth now and gave up your job, because the work you're doing will only get more difficult with time and worsen in quality. You could end up being fired and lose your disability insurance." Louis was aghast. "Your day has come. Work is over for you, Louis, but life isn't." I could see the realization wash over his body like a tidal wave; he knew I was right. Louis didn't cry that day, or even tear up, he just stared blankly at the floor for what seemed an eternity. He looked up, he would give up, he would quit work. But he would not quit living.

To this day Louis remains thankful for our arrival that afternoon. Before that hour, it wasn't in his consciousness to give up work. He was struggling with how to function in the face of stumbling concentration and faltering skills, and he was losing the fight. To reach a point of understanding the necessity for this drastic change, the input of others can quiet the noise. It's easier, of course, to bring another person to that place of loss once you've been there yourself. I could help him see the truth; I had been there myself. In many ways, I still am.

LOST IN A WHISPER

John Embry and I didn't see much of each other, although occasionally we would get together with other friends for dinner. Then I met Lance and he and I made the move to San Francisco. After the move whenever Lance and I visited L.A. we would drop in on John, but I saw him less and less as our trips south became fewer. On one of these trips, however, Lance was occupied and so I called John to go out to the bars with me, like we had done in the past. Soon we were standing around talking small stuff. Neither of us mentioned the many we had known who were now gone. But we were both quiet as I drove John home that night. When we arrived at his apartment, I got out of my car to hug him. As he walked up the little hill to where he lived he spoke without turning around,

"They're just shells, you know. That's all that's left."

Almost certainly he spoke of our bodies—the cocoons we live in now—which are buried or burned when we die. I'll never know his subtleties of reflection as I didn't stop him to ask. That was the last time I saw him.

I hadn't seen John for several years when Hurricane Katrina hit New Orleans in 2005. I saw, as did everyone, the TV reports of the devastation and lack of medical personnel. Although I was rusty, I volunteered to serve with the Red Cross in any capacity except as a physician or nurse. I thought I could be of service even if just a body far from the "glamorous" epicenter in New Orleans—in Dallas, say, or Atlanta. I truthfully told them I had AIDS, and to ensure I was a help and not a hinderance my star of a partner (not yet husband), Frank, offered to pay for the airline ticket and any hotel costs, as well as watch over me. I attended a Red Cross class for voluntary medical personnel and, unlike me, emailed my plans to a short list of people close to me. John responded immediately with a return message saying the Red Cross would be lucky to have me—even as a rusty medical doctor with AIDS.

The Red Cross, even with my medical volunteer training, subsequently turned me down and I licked my wounds. More months than I care to admit passed without John and I communicating. One night I was on the phone with a mutual friend of ours, Bill Litts, when he mentioned in passing John's death. I was surprised, but not shocked, to hear that he had died. When had he passed away? Of what had he died? Bill couldn't help; he didn't know any details. I called another mutual friend, but that friend's phone had been disconnected—another friend gone missing in the age of HIV. I damned myself for not keeping in touch although it would have been contrary to one of my rules of the plague: you didn't keep in contact with people unless you and they had been extraordinarily close. But John had meant much to me and my resistance to attachment had been to my painful disadvantage.

He'd been so faithful in holding friends tightly and yet my last visit with him had been rushed and short. In spite of my education and training, it was John who had been the most forceful in showing me the need to stay close to friends. All the flat surfaces in his house had been crowded with photographs of his friends—both living and dead. He had kept a picture of my Jack in his living room and, indeed, had attended his funeral Mass. In these years, protease inhibitors or not, friendships had to be constantly cultivated, connections had to be maintained. Or they were gone in a moment, lost in a whisper.

MARK HIGGINS, M.D.—
"CONDUITS OF HEALING"

Mark Higgins, M.D., my extraordinary physician, reports a patient who lost his partner of 11 years to AIDS. The following year this HIV-negative man found himself compelled to end a budding relationship in large part due to that person's HIV status. This gentleman readily admitted that he couldn't support this decision morally or politically, but he simply couldn't put himself in the position of caretaker again. He couldn't be what Dr. Higgins calls a "conduit of healing." I've felt the same emotional turmoil. Those of us who lived through this period have experienced something very rare—on occasion we've had to let laboratory findings veto relationships.

Mark acknowledged that we can't always be messengers of relief, but added that our inability to always live up to our own sometimes impossibly high standards can't be something we carry guilt about. We can't help everyone all the time. We're only human and there are times when we must also nurture ourselves. An army can't go to war unless it's fed and clothed. Although I'm loathe to say it, perhaps this should color our thinking at least a little when we are tempted to judge our brothers on the occasions when we see what appears to be cowardice or desertion. On those occasions when we see someone who appears to be taking the easy way out, perhaps we should wonder how well their soldiers are fed and their army clothed.

That being said, there are still some times when our internal compass tells us that our actions and understanding are not enough. We feel self-reproach for not being there for a loved one in his time of need or for going on to experience years of life after a loved one is gone. These are some of the bruises and lacerations of "survivor's

ANDREW M. FAULK, M.D.

guilt." I wrestle with the regret of not having been a better friend, not having had more patience, not saying aloud what my heart felt... guilt that I wasn't a better person. Times when I suddenly suck air into my lungs when stumbling upon a memory. Moments when I wonder if my troops could've fought harder, longer, with what they had.

STAYING AWAY FROM THE TAKE-AWAYS

So why wasn't I absolutely devastated by the scope and speed of the demolition of our community? I was scared, no doubt about it. But not to the point of paralysis. A part of me was watching what was going on and saying, "Oh, yes, is this how it's going to be? This quick?" And I think speed isn't an enemy. After I had left the practice, Fred Lawrence and I spoke infrequently, but on one occasion we discussed the death of one of our patients who was a famous Walt Disney lyricist. He lived in New York, but sometimes came to LMG for a second opinion and information on possible new medications. He had passed away just before he had won several national and international awards. I asked Fred, isn't it an incredible shame this man died, right when all these good things were about to happen for him? Fred responded that, to the contrary, it was a perfect time for him to die—right when the world was at his fingertips, when he was at that exquisite moment when he was anticipating phenomenal success. What a great time to die! I don't know that I can sign on to this assessment.

To this day, when I hear the lyrics of one of his iconic theme songs, I weep, immediately. Sometimes I believe I'm wearing internal bifocals: one part frightened by the future, one part interested in how it will play out. When the take-aways come however—especially when they want to take away my car keys—it will be a very dark day.

ANDREW M. FAULK, M.D.

FIGHTING GRAVITY

As life moves on, I find that I imagine myself similar to an unsuccessful space shuttle that shudders more and more intensely, and then explodes as it re-enters the earth's atmosphere. Deficiencies of the body are such that it will not survive the re-entry process as it encounters the friction and force of the earth's atmosphere. It shakes and tumbles as it hurtles toward destruction. In spite of the life-saving cocktail of medications, I feel that in a similar way the vehicle of my body sustains increasing neurologic degeneration and white cell destruction as the disease progresses to its inevitable conclusion. And at present I cope with the shocks and turbulence as best I can, all the while trying to enjoy the ride.

"PINK SATURDAY"—
PARTY DAY BEFORE PRIDE PARADE

On June 27, 2009, Dick Bretto had a Pink Saturday get-together with a few guests, one of them being Stan Ridge of Arizona. "Pink Saturdays" are the Saturday evenings before Gay Pride Sunday. When I was still in practice in LMG, Stan made the trip from Arizona every few months to see me. The cornerstone of his personality is calm, measured logic. I don't remember if his status had been discovered with me, but if it had he certainly didn't exhibit histrionics. He's the sort of person who takes such information in stride, acknowledging the natural fear, but quickly moving on to the next step, whatever it may be. In many ways, he reminded me of myself—logic told him what's done is done and the goal was to be happy and fulfilled, despite any possible impending catastrophe.

By the time he walked into my exam room in 1990 more was known, paradoxically, about how little we knew. And with that knowledge came insight into the awful limitations of medicine. We could prescribe AZT, but little else. In a short amount of time, however, the tools of Pentamidine and later Septra for PCP prophylaxis would come. But for that particular time, it was not only logical, but also calming to concede the limitations of medicine and live daily in that acceptance. As someone living with HIV and knowing I was doing what little could be done, I was free to live life without constant worry and fear. What would happen, would happen. It was an era of making the best of one's time. Stan's visits were matter-of-fact and even serene especially because his disease wasn't progressing by the metrics at hand.

At the time, my personal HIV status was not discussed with any of my patients, including Stan. Would a hospital, insurance provider, or senior physician be accountable if an HIV-positive doctor were to disclose the fact? I had found myself out of one closet only to find myself in another. But living quietly, below radar, was second nature. Dr. John Gamble at CPMC had never known my status, saving him the potential storm of cutting me off from patient contact. Neither Fred nor Vincent knew I was HIV-positive, and Stan naturally didn't ask. Before President Clinton's precipitous armed services policy, physicians with HIV were already living in a "Don't Ask, Don't Tell" world.

When I left my practice I told Stan of my disease. So now on Pink Saturday some two decades later, he and I stood looking down Castro Street from its junction with Market Street, with hundreds of jubilant gay and lesbian party revelers. We stood, side by side, our hands resting on each other's hip. "It's so great that we're here, that we both have survived to see this together," I said.

"Yes, it's really phenomenal," he said as we gave each other a hug.

THE MAGIC JOHNSON MOMENT

Today is Michael Jackson's funeral, and as I watch Earvin "Magic" Johnson give his eulogy there, I am reminded of when he surrendered his basketball career on November 7, 1991, after announcing he was HIV-positive (after long denying he had "the AIDS disease"). No doubt he made his decision in the belief, shared by so many of us, that his life was soon to end and duplicity in keeping such a secret from a sensationalism-loving public would have been onerous, and in the end, unsuccessful. But the overflowing of acceptance and good will by the general public was met with bitterness by many of my gay brothers—bitterness toward a public which, before a celebrity's mention, had shown so little concern or even acknowledgment, of this disease which had felled thousands of us.

I had begun participating in an HIV-positive group of health care professionals several months before Jack's death. Actually, I only learned the group was of HIV-positive health care workers the first time I attended. I had signed up on the advice of a colleague for what I thought was merely a group of health care professionals working with HIV-positive patients, not necessarily for health care providers who were HIV-positive themselves. While it was an important distinction, as I was no longer in practice its relevance had vanished. My support group felt not just resentment but outright anger toward this outpouring of sympathy for the celebrity Magic Johnson. "Now, suddenly, they've heard of HIV. Now, now that somebody famous and likable has contracted HIV, somebody 'sympathetic,' they see us? How many people have died and they're just discovering it now?"

To me it is a mere technicality that President Ronald Reagan, "The Great Communicator," finally spoke about AIDS in May,

ANDREW M. FAULK, M.D.

1987—until that time he hadn't uttered the word in public. At that point 36,058 Americans had been diagnosed with AIDS and 20,849 had died (approximately 58,000 Americans died in the Vietnam War). In the following years his lack of leadership was deadly—it rationalized minuscule research funding and fueled mainstream fear and hatred of gay men. The activist-author Larry Kramer has written that he "murdered more gay people than anyone in the entire history of the world." Reagan's indifference reinforced the hostile zealotry of Christian Evangelicals such as Jerry Falwell, who preached that "AIDS was the wrath of God on homosexuals." Indeed Reagan's Communications Director, Pat Buchanan, stated that AIDS was "nature's revenge on gay men."

Thus the epidemic was compounded by a society which left us and our dying brothers largely abandoned and without services from kitchens to mortuaries. To their great credit it was the lesbian community as well as that of many heterosexual groups such as pockets of Catholic charities—after their rejection of papal rules and sensibilities—that jumped in to orchestrate AIDS fundraising, education and, that mark of true dedication and self-sacrifice, one-on-one care. They were the ones who, led by their sense of active compassion, began and staffed hospices, ran food delivery services to the house-bound and held the hand of the dying when their families shunned them. AIDS was devastating to the gay community and its supporters but, on the other hand, it frequently minimized our differences and bettered the world of the poor and sick.

DOPPELGÄNGERS OF GRIEF

There were occasions when we would be someplace—perhaps a grocery store, a restaurant—and we would notice the back of someone's head, the way he stood, or the side of his face. A breath would catch in our throat. Is it him? We couldn't help ourselves; we would move closer for a better look. Then our stomach would drop. No, of course it wasn't him, and we would quickly look away in a twinge of embarrassment.

Or we would feel someone looking at us—in that way of possible recognition. Were we, their love, now dead? How could this be?

This experience was repeated, multiplied, over and over again. Gay men got used to certain looks or being approached, with sidelong glasses, by a stranger because they understood that they bore some resemblance to the missing. All of us, the children of Hamelin, got used to being mistaken for that loved one. It may not have mattered to the one viewed, but the terrible wound reopened by such collision would ache the heart once more.

Sometimes this encounter with a *doppelgänger* of grief would graduate to an introduction of sorts. But the sorrow would remain.

ANDREW M. FAULK, M.D.

MY PARTNERSHIP WITH FRANK

Frank Jernigan and I began dating in 2004 when he was living in a one-room studio filled with orchids and an elderly cocker spaniel. He was a fascinating man: compassionate, brilliant and, I was eventually to learn, tremendously generous. Frank was unlike anyone I had ever met.

His life had not followed any ordinary trajectory. After being a self-described "Jesus Freak" in Berkeley in the hippie years of 1969 and '70, he married a deeply spiritual woman, Karolyn, with whom he has two daughters. He went on to pastor churches in Maine and Massachusetts and eventually came out to the world—and himself— at the age of 43. Karolyn and he divorced, out of necessity rather than antipathy. But the home-church they helped found was disinclined to choose love and humility over dogma and summarily asked Frank to leave. It is the nature and history of our family to be at remarkable peace with each other—thus Karolyn has become a good friend of mine. In 2000, after years studying computer engineering, Frank moved from Boston to San Francisco for the Dot-Com Boom which soon became the Dot-Com Bust. Applying to different computer companies, he was hired by Google at the age of 55—a company famous for the youth of its employees.

It was early in our relationship when Frank invited me to the 2004 Google Christmas party. When he suggested I wear a suit, I took it more seriously than he intended. Neither having one nor the time to buy one new, I descended on my local secondhand outlet with a frenzy borne of desperation. Although I found a suit, it was disturbingly too large and I threw myself on the mercy of an untried, although handy, neighborhood tailor. Having given him as much time as possible, I returned only to discover my suit augmented rather than diminished! With only hours to go, I should have opted for needle, thread, and a few surgeon's knots. Instead, I reached for my stapler. That night I was to discover that staples itch ferociously.

The Google engineers were oblivious to my ongoing discomfort which only entertained Frank the more.

He is now my legal husband—an officially-recognized relationship inconceivable in earlier years. For gay couples multiple anniversaries are not uncommon and, fortunately or unfortunately, they provide opportunities for both celebration and memory failure. We were initially married in our backyard in 2007 and then legally in San Francisco City Hall on November 4, 2008. An historically inauspicious day, that November 4 was the election day when the infamous Proposition 8 passed which suspended further same-sex marriages in California. Like others of that period, however, our marriage remained valid throughout the ensuing legal battles and is legally recognized today.

One of Frank's daughters, Sadie Valeri, has become an internationally-recognized painter in the classical realism style, while her husband, Nowell, is a music composer and video producer. Frank's youngest daughter, Angela, is a Minister in the United Church of Christ and a parent educator; she and her husband, Niels Teunis, an anthropologist, have our one grandchild, Leah. Never having had children, it's quite a shock to find oneself a grandfather!

For the first time in my life I have a long-term relationship with someone without HIV, and Frank has remained so throughout our years together. Having come out later in life, Frank never experienced being a 23-year-old waiting in line outside some club wearing tight pants and a T-shirt at midnight in the pouring rain. He never was the young, gym-obsessed, fashion-conscious, urban, gay male. Nor has he suffered the brunt of a horrific avalanche of friends and lovers developing AIDS and dying. He has largely lived several degrees removed from HIV and the turbulence it brought to the gay community—which is gratifying and disconcerting at the same time. When I was in the turmoil of my practice, I presumed that life for our society could never, ever be the same—that it never, ever *should* be the same. But Frank's world didn't experience such heart-breaking, catastrophic upheavals—his has been a different universe. While I more than occasionally feel the solitude of my illness, I celebrate his escape. And though he's not as familiar with AIDS as he might be, we married when we both knew I had AIDS. Many HIV-negative men would have declined such a marriage, knowing the possibility that their husband might well face this savage assassin. Had our positions be reversed, I myself would have thought long and hard. In fact, I believe I would have declined. Instead he opened his heart and allowed our relationship to flourish, and so it has changed my life.

These days his isolation from the disease is no longer what it was. My day-to-day life is punctuated by occasional episodes of what he and I call my "Swiss cheese" memory—unpredictable "holes" in my short-term recollection. I frequently become irritated with Frank for his assuming I remember something I don't or for assuming I don't remember something I do. But how can he predict what I'll recall and what I won't? My memory is not the only thing which makes life perplexing: my speech disorder is occasionally overwhelming, my balance and tremor worrisome. I tire easily and find it exhausting to be around people for long periods of time. But throughout these thorny difficulties Frank has proven himself a loving partner.

FRANK'S VISITS TO SAN QUENTIN

It is Frank's understanding that much happiness comes from improving the lives of others and he works to help those whose help is most needed. Before he retired Frank established a foundation for the advancement of human well-being. Every December we Jernigans assemble to happily choose various groups and individuals to be recipients of the Jernigan Charitable Foundation. While the Foundation's contributions are deeply satisfying, Frank's efforts have not been limited to financial donations. One of his acquaintances, Nicola Bucci, was a chef at Google who was in a terrible car accident that happened without the involvement of alcohol or drugs. In 2008 he was wrongly convicted of Second-Degree Murder and sentenced to 23 years to life; he presently is an inmate in San Quentin State Prison. While others have ignored Bucci and his situation, Frank has worked tirelessly for his release. He has contacted the State Attorney General's office, written letters to US Representative Nancy Pelosi and other congress-persons as well as the ACLU. Frank visits Bucci in San Quentin every weekend but, as part of the "hoops" he has to jump through, he must make a pre-visit request two weeks in advance and then, at the prison, wait for an hour and a half and go through two security examinations. Bucci is never far from Frank's mind—we've been in London and he has taken the time to visit people who knew Bucci and perhaps could help with his case. While Bucci may have been forgotten by his old friends and society at large, he hasn't been forgotten by Frank.

"Spiritual" is a word Frank rarely uses, but he earns it every day just the same.

THE CHAIR UPHOLSTERED IN MEMORIES

We have room on the first floor of our house here in Noe Valley for the things we don't have room for elsewhere. The blending of furniture naturally occurs when a couple moves in together and a rose-colored winged chair of mine finally found a home here on the first level. Last night my eye caught a bit of tag hanging from its bottom carriage that I hadn't seen before and which had no doubt surfaced in the chaos of cleaning. The tag is the "customer reference" slip showing the chair's date of order as 5/16/91 and its "scheduled ship date" as 6/14/91—10 days after Jack's death.

During that last year of Jack's life there were the usual multiple hospitalizations which accompany the diagnosis of AIDS and cancer, and I was scurrying to find distractions to keep his mind occupied and his spirits up. One of these diversions was ordering this winged chair that now stands as mute reminder of those days. Years before I had sat next to Jack's bed and placing the order for this chair drew our attention away from the walls of his room in UCLA Hospital and became a happy focus. I remember our choosing the color there, and the fabric design. That day had been a lighter day—like the framed posters I hung in his room each hospitalization, as a way of giving him something on which to focus as well as bring something non-institutional into his room. These posters—as bits of our home—were visual reminders of his latest survival. The winged chair, with its comfort of enclosing arms, did the same, if not more.

MY WORST NIGHTMARE

Since being in practice, a particular nightmare has haunted me more than any other. It is not the most frequent but it is arguably the most disturbing. When I have dreamt it, I have been known to talk in my sleep (unusual for me) and when I awaken I am upset and depressed throughout the ensuing day. When it first began in 1990 I experienced it once a week or so, now I'm relieved to have it only about twice a year.

I'm in a darkened warehouse directly underneath one harsh solitary light. Parked askew from each other are two trucks which are nearly identical. I see very little of their cabs, but they're old-fashioned and their beds, being without roofs, are constructed with wooden sides and wooden floors.

In the dream I am pulling large crates, one at a time, from one truck bed and pushing them onto the floor of the other. The movement of these boxes produces a loud scraping sound which breaks a dead silence. My efforts are steady, but the work isn't particularly tiring and the pace is manageable. In the world outside our dreams, I would be unable to perform this task due to the size and weight of these objects but in dreams, as we know, there are no such limitations. In the first months I experienced the dream, I would load and unload them without notice or knowledge of their grim contents—the horrifying awareness of exactly what I was carrying would evolve only gradually. In the years following, by contrast, I have immediately known what these boxes were and my dreadful work.

For they are not simply crates, they are coffins.

And this terrible vision is magnified by the fact they are not ordinary coffins—they are caskets made of glass. I can clearly see

ANDREW M. FAULK, M.D.

into and through all of them. Each one has within it a corpse: a figure which is visible, a body which I can see. Emaciated and horribly disfigured by KS lesions, the cadavers shift and rock from the motion of my work. These are my brothers.

More disturbing than the gruesome setting is my mission. This is the crux of my nightmare—more than the bodies I see is the awareness that I'm fundamentally powerless against the juggernaut of HIV. In the real world I could treat some of the opportunistic illnesses which HIV presents along the way, but in my dream I'm merely transferring patients' remains from one location to another—I'm rearranging chairs on the deck of the Titanic. I can't affect the slaughter and the understanding washes over me as forcefully as a tidal wave, sucking my breath away and drowning me in its undertow.

SURVIVOR'S GUILT

Until I die I will face a burden of guilt which cannot be detached from my survival. If I could separate the confusing feelings of grief and guilt I carry, I would be more able to cope with each. But I don't experience them in tidy, discrete packages. Instead I experience swirls of emotions which flow into and out of each other creating a painful and bewildering maelstrom. Grief is one thing, guilt is quite another, but it can be difficult for me to distinguish where one begins and the other ends. Unless I am vigilant in policing my thoughts with consciousness and logic, the two combine to form a whole bigger than their parts.

The most powerful guilt I feel comes from my survival during a time when those who died and those who didn't seems monstrously random. I live with the haunting sensation that I should have died along with my brothers. Guilt is deserved blame, but here the blame is undeserved and this false culpability, manufactured from the underlying sense that in my survival somehow lies the deaths of my peers, presumes a zero-sum situation—a circumstance in which should someone live, I die; if I should live than another dies. Sometimes my self-esteem stumbles and I face accusation arising from the warped perception that many of these deaths are of people I judge to be better than I. And blame cascades onto more blame as I gauge their lives as impacting the world more than that of my own. Such thinking, however, is neither logical nor legitimate: my value is as great, of course, as any other. But my guilt from surviving rises and falls from time to time, situation to situation, memory to memory. When a bullet misses you and kills the one standing next to you, are you to blame? What if the one killed next to you is your best

ANDREW M. FAULK, M.D.

friend? Your lover? I must continually remind myself that there is no fault in survival—the perpetuation of my life does not cut another man's short. I am innocent of the deaths of those around me.

Having been a physician during the plague I also am painfully battered, at times, by the thought that if I had only done *more* for my patients, they would be alive today. These people were in my care. They were my responsibility and they died. How can I not bear some blame for their deaths? Had I sacrificed more, somehow, would fewer of my patients have died? Throughout the day I walk with ghosts and at 3 a.m. my share of responsibility for their deaths feels monumental.

We now have the anti-viral cocktail and HIV is more manageable, yet I am hounded by the sense that in some parallel universe in which time is inconstant, the medications of today were available in the past but unused with terrible consequence. This is not a rational imagination, but I *feel* it just the same. The truth of that time was that we could treat an infection or condition here and there, but it was a never-ending case of winning the battle but losing the war.

Yet our only shortcomings were those of medical science, not training or dedication. We did all that we could with the tools that we had.

There is another type of guilt distinct from that described above, derived from what I did and didn't do in the non-medical realm. When I think of Jack and the many I loved, I can easily bury myself in a blizzard of regrets for those acts I didn't do, efforts I didn't make, and qualities I didn't have. Why didn't I do this or say that? Did I provide all the emotional support I could? Did I fail those near me during what remained of their time on earth? There are times when this blame is the most heavy of them all.

Today as I navigate my course through eddies of grief and blame, I strive to keep in mind the worth of my brothers and the courage of their struggle without assuming the self-reproach that I, too, should have passed away. I harbor blame for the failures I made with those I loved, but I must forgive myself—for to forgive is to release. And there exists little benefit in holding tightly to the past. Living my life as fully as I can and as happily as I am able does not corrupt my innocence. Those that have passed away were people whose lives illuminate and inform my own to this day and I do them no disrespect by living without regret or recrimination.

CONFRONTING DEATH

Sometimes I'm able to "accept" my death, at least that's the wording that comes the most easily to me. But it's not my death I struggle with but rather the heartache I experience in the anticipation of the all-encompassing loss of myself—the annihilation of all those millions of memories and idiosyncrasies, thoughts and feelings, that are unique to me and make up who I am. To paraphrase Clint Eastwood's character in the film *Unforgiven*, "death takes away not only what you have, but everything you'll ever have," while the philosopher Heidigger more precisely describes death as "the impossibility of further possibility." The greater truth that supersedes the glib is that what I battle is not fear of being dead but rather the despair of losing a future.

I don't deal with the anguish of that impending loss as a one-time event, position or even journey. I slip and slide through the Kübler-Ross stages of grief—denial, anger, bargaining, depression and, yes, acceptance. I approach these different plateaus at different times and frequently revisit those with which I have previously struggled. I question myself—am I moving on to another stage or am I revisiting one I thought I had reconciled? It seems I can manage the anguish in one moment and be far from comforted the next. The place where I spend most of my time and energy, however, is in that state of "modified denial": I don't take notice that I have a disease, but I swallow my medications and visit my doctors just the same. But even this one form of denial isn't and can't be permanent.

The existential kernel of death, it seems to me, is transiency. Philosophical Buddhism focuses on the temporary nature of all material things and, indeed, of life itself. When I intellectually grasp

ANDREW M. FAULK, M.D.

this impermanence and feel it, I realize the way to love anyone or experience anything with the greatest depth is to be aware that all things are passing and destined to be lost. At the end of the film *Blade Runner*, the narrator notes that in the last few moments of the artificial human's life, when the "replicant" poignantly comprehends the fragility of life and the approaching destruction of everything that makes him an individual, that is when he loves life the most. When I'm aware of the passing nature of life I find myself in contact with the passion and depth of living but also—in that awareness—I connect with the serenity of accepting the fleeting nature of reality as natural and inevitable. Yet to live in this emotional perception from moment to moment I find difficult and intermittent.

I realize that many whom I envy believe death doesn't result in oblivion but rather eternal presence and serenity. I know these people enjoy an equanimity which helps them achieve longer and less troubled lives. I wish I had such beliefs; but no matter how motivated, I can't believe in an after-life. When I attempt to believe in a God, I have the overpowering feeling I'm just fooling myself—as if I were trying to convince myself to believe a placebo was true medicine. I can't embrace philosophies which deny the laws of nature in favor of, what is for me, intellectual anarchy. If I could, my life would be easier. Yet the story of my gentleman who experienced a near-death experience argues in favor of the spiritual world of which I am so skeptical. These two explanations, spiritual and scientific, defy integration which leaves me stranded with a dramatic and muscular cognitive dissonance.

Jack lacked the surety of eternal life and couldn't acknowledge his coming end; the last day of his life he asked for the details of our future medical strategy. Recognition is necessary for acceptance and as he didn't concede his end he escaped the greater battle. His partner previous to me, Ted, was a man I never met. But evidently, after the epidemic exploded, Ted became hypochondriac—his realization of the disease with which he was living produced constant fear that any cough or lesion was the beginning of a death spiral. If anything, stress itself can cause full-blown AIDS to develop more quickly. I knew many men who had adopted Ted's response and spent their remaining weeks in the same emotional chaos—in the end his fears eclipsed his happiness and wasted precious energy.

It's no surprise that my daily struggles with the recognition of my coming extinction produce an awareness of transiency which increasingly draws me in to a way to deal with the sorrow of impending death and, surprisingly, provides a route to happiness. I may dislike the phenomenon, but I know by experience and research that happiness doesn't correlate with wealth in achievement or goods. I imagine I'll be happy if I become this or obtain that, but once I've attained this position or acquired that item, my happiness becomes tied to yet another goal or object, and so keeps drifting out of reach. With the comprehension of my impending death, however, the value of the present becomes tangible. And this awareness that all I see and feel, every object and moment, is destined for oblivion makes me love all those bits and pieces of life all the more and I am propelled into loving the present more than fearing the future.

ANDREW M. FAULK, M.D.

NATIONAL MARCH STIRS MEMORIES:
WE SHALL OVERCOME

At the 2009 National Equality March on Washington, D.C., Stan Ridge, a former patient of mine, and Frank and I are introduced to Trudy Shepard, the mother of Matthew Shepard, who was tortured and murdered in Wyoming in 1998.

* * *

In the spring of 1987, there came a time when it was necessary to conference with a family on how aggressive to be with the care of an AIDS patient near death in CPMC's ICU. His mother, sister and brother had flown in from the Midwest while our patient, having pulmonary KS, was *in extremis* on a ventilator. While we could possibly lengthen his life by a week or two, longer than that was very doubtful and we needed instructions on how aggressively to treat him. The family listened quietly, although the sister fidgeted constantly. She was not in the healthcare field and her questions showed that she was out of her depth. Each time we mentioned one of the possibilities that could lead to patient improvement, the sister became more agitated. Finally the question she had been wanting to ask surfaced: "Can't we do something to hurry his death along?" We were stunned. It fell to Dr. Ron Elkin, the ICU Attending, to respond and we waited for his answer. Ron was a very low-keyed person but we saw his eyes widen with her question. Before he could reply, she continued that she had flown out to San Francisco leaving her job behind and needed to return by office hours on Monday. She needed to get back to work.

Ron responded that "hurrying things along" was not only ethically unconscionable but legally questionable. She stated matter-of-factly, "Well, you're doctors, aren't you?"

"That isn't what we do," he answered flatly.

She was obviously disappointed with this response. "Well, I have to be back by Monday, you all need to decide what to do," she stood up and walked out of the room. By the following Monday she was indeed back at her job. Her brother had passed.

* * *

David Mixner, civil rights activist and author, spoke at the National March and choked up when he spoke of parents not willing to visit a gay son in the hospital. Once rounding on a sleeping LMG patient in the Medical Center of North Hollywood, I noticed an opened greeting card standing up on our patient's tray table. I knew little about this particular patient as he was routinely seen by Vincent or Fred. It may have been improper, but I picked up the Hallmark card which on the face was printed something painfully unrealistic about wishing he got well soon. On the inside, across from some printed message equally as vacuous as that on the front, was a handwritten note, "Peter, we know that if you would just repent from your sins, and ask Jesus into your heart, God will heal you. As long as you continue living in sin, though, we don't feel right coming to visit." It was signed "Mother."

Peter died the following week.

* * *

There at the National Equality March on Washington, I looked at the huge crowd and thought, we have all lived with this burden our entire lives. We have been judged, excluded and made to pay a price for the differences in our natural hearts, and for abandoning suffocating closets. But it's only time before we win our freedoms and rights and, I have no doubt, acceptance. My father already accepts me and has grieved over his past treatment of me—one day America will do the same. This resolute understanding was woven into the fabric of the demonstration and its unifying theme: "We shall overcome."

ANDREW M. FAULK, M.D.

A SURVIVOR

It's been 30 years since I was in that exam room receiving the worst news of my life. Although my generation was decimated by HIV, I have survived the epidemic. The certainty of my imminent death was mistaken, for these days most HIV patients die from something other than AIDS. The medical difficulties and many medications I take, as well as underlying limitations and isolation are significant, but they are manageable. They are, as they say, the "cost of doing business."

There's an old word in German for the advanced education one receives from serious illness: *Siechtumsschulung*. From my long struggle with HIV, I've developed certain goals that, while not necessarily realized, are clear. The most important objective I've found is mindfulness—the awareness of where I am and what I'm doing in any given moment. The immutable past and the unknowable future can drain attention away from the most important piece of time we have—the present. When we live in the moment, we're more likely to act in it and more likely to ensure that those we love know they're cherished. Continuing awareness of the possibility of a sudden end doesn't have to mean living in fear of the future, but rather it can serve as powerful motivation to live more fully in the present and with focused attention.

I've learned happiness is an accomplishment more than a condition. Many of my brothers, when pushed to their absolute limit and in incredible distress, chose a road which led to a better place than where they began—a place of giving and forgiveness. Living with the possibility of coming pain and loss of control has taught me that happiness can often be found in simple, uncomplicated activities. That it's easier for happiness to occur when I live in a spirit of gratitude. That I can relax knowing that worry burns precious energy, for I can do what I can do and no more.

My work was extraordinarily difficult—not just in intellectual challenge, but also in emotional demand. I discovered, however, a transcendent meaning in work which occurs when we serve a purpose beyond ourselves, for a meaningful life is more satisfying than merely a happy life. It became apparent to me that we can achieve a consciousness of overriding significance when we focus attention away from ourselves and towards others; there is a unique satisfaction which comes from this redirection.

Siechtumsschulung, if nothing else, has taught me priorities in terms of perception and thought. While it's still a challenge to maintain my equilibrium in the face of consequential incidents and accidents, I've discovered it's rarely difficult to deal with the trinkets of disappointment and aggravation we all encounter daily. I'm no longer completely invested in a particular result—for example in conversation with Frank, he or I may comment on a desired event or hoped-for result, and then one of us will say "or not." We may be passionate about an outcome, but we're also prepared for it to end differently than we'd like.

Having acquired a measure of *Siechtumsschulung*, I hope that when my time comes for that walk off the earth, the courage and serenity of so many of my brothers will surface in me. That I'll reject the poison of self-pity and continue to fight for what is possible in the midst of what is not. Struggle and surrender, intermixed.

I believe that in remembering the bright and the beautiful lost to this, the greatest plague in generations, we not only do them honor but also acknowledge that the work found in helping dying people face their end has its own value—its own success in unsuccessful times. When it comes to so many of my friends who have died I can say I gave the best friendship I was able. And for my patients who, almost to a person, have passed, I rest in certain confidence that I did my best to treat their disease and gently prepare them for approaching death. A quote I treasure says "People may not remember exactly what you did, or what you said, but they will always remember how you made them feel. Remember, what you do echoes in eternity." My hope is that how I made my patients feel will echo throughout eternity.

ANDREW M. FAULK, M.D.

Donations to support AIDS research may be sent to the University of Washington.

ANDREW M. FAULK, M.D.
ENDOWED FUND FOR HIV/AIDS

UNIVERSITY OF WASHINGTON SCHOOL OF MEDICINE

Gifts can be made to the Andrew M. Faulk, M.D. Endowed Fund for HIV/AIDS by searching for that fund on this page:

https://www.washington.edu/giving/make-a-gift

Gifts by check may be made out to "Andrew M. Faulk, M.D. Endowed Fund" and sent to:

UW Medicine Advancement
Attn: Gift Processing
Box 358045
Seattle, WA 98195-8045